D1578509

Clinical anatomy fo

Clinical anatomy
for dentistry

Richard B. Longmore BSc, BDS, PhD
General Dental Practitioner; formerly Senior Lecturer in
Anatomy, University of Dundee, Dundee, UK

Duncan A. McRae MB ChB
Registrar in Psychiatry, Royal Dundee Liff Hospital; formerly
Lecturer in Anatomy, University of Dundee, Dundee, UK

CHURCHILL LIVINGSTONE
EDINBURGH LONDON MELBOURNE AND NEW YORK 1985

CHURCHILL LIVINGSTONE
Medical Division of Longman Group Limited

Distributed in the United States of America by Churchill
Livingstone Inc., 1560 Broadway, New York, N.Y. 10036, and
by associated companies, branches and representatives
throughout the world.

First published/1985

ISBN 0 443 02573 8

British Library Cataloguing in Publication Data

Longmore, R.B.
    Clinical anatomy for dentistry. — (Dental series)
    1. Face   2. Jaws
    I. Title   II. McRae, D.A.   III. Series
    612'.92   QM535

Library of Congress Cataloging in Publication Data

Longmore, R. B.
    Clinical anatomy for dentistry.

    1. Head — Anatomy.   2. Neck — Anatomy.   3.
    Dentistry.
    I. McRae, D. A.   II. Title.   [DNLM: 1. Dentistry.
    2. Head — anatomy & histology.   3. Neck — anatomy &
    Histology.   WU 101 L856c]
    RK280.L65   1985   611'.91   84-23770

Produced by Longman Singapore Publishers Pte Ltd
Printed in Singapore.

To our wives
Mary Longmore and Janice McRae
with love and thanks

Preface

Dentistry involves the diagnosis, prevention and treatment of oral disease. The clinical appearance and subsequent behaviour of oral disease is governed by anatomical and physiological factors which can also modify the method of treatment.

Dentistry is an intensely practical discipline. In the undergraduate curriculum much emphasis is given to the acquisition of manual skills. This may be at the expense of a thorough understanding of the anatomical, physiological and biochemical basis of the clinical conditions concerned. It is understandably difficult for someone studying anatomy to see the relevance of aged, embalmed and invariably edentulous cadavers to clinical dentistry. This text is intended to stress to the pre-clinical and clinical student, and to the qualified practitioner, that an understanding of anatomy is relevant and important in clinical dentistry. It is neither a detailed textbook of anatomy nor does it encompass all aspects of clinical dentistry. The text should be read in conjunction with more detailed books of anatomy and clinical dentistry and with the study of the living tissues in patients, contemporaries or self.

Diagnosis has two components: the taking of a *case-history* and the *clinical examination* of the patient. The case-history is taken by interview with the patient, and the *symptoms* which have prompted the consultation are recorded. A symptom is an alteration in the structure or function of some part or parts of the body, for example, 'my gums have swollen and bleed easily'. A *medical history* is taken to discover whether there are any factors which might influence dental treatment or be a contributing factor to the patients symptoms. A *dental history* is taken to record the types of dental treatment received in the past, particularly any complications or difficulties that arose from it.

Clinical examination has two parts. *Observation* of the patient should commence *before* the history is taken. Factors such as the demeanour, gait and behaviour should be noted on first encountering the patient. *Physical examination* of the patient should be systematic. Extraoral examination by observation and palpation should note the facial expression, which may denote a disturbed emotional state, texture and colour of the skin and any facial asymmetry or swelling. Mandibular posture and movements, together with the temporomandibular joints, should be examined. Lymph nodes of the head and neck should be examined methodically, including the deep cervical chain. *Intraorally*, the oral mucosa, including the gingiva, should be examined with particular reference to its colour, texture and the presence of swellings or ulceration. The teeth present should be recorded and examined for abnormalities, tenderness and mobility.

A *provisional diagnosis* is then made. This may be precise, for example, a carious tooth which explains the patient's symptoms of pain. In some instances, e.g. an atypical facial pain, a variety of conditions may be thought likely to explain the symptoms. Further examinations are carried out and these can include radiological, microbiological, haematological, biochemical and histopathological investigations.

A *final diagnosis* of the condition or conditions producing the patient's symptoms is made and an appropriate course of treatment, if agreed by the patient, is then carried out.

The successful clinical examination particularly

requires that the clinician can detect abnormalities from the *normal* in the behaviour, structure and function of tissues. An understanding of the normal is therefore essential for the practice of clinical dentistry.

Dundee, 1985   R.B.L
                                                D.A.M.

Contents

Development and structure of the dental tissues

TEETH

Structure (Fig. 1.1)

Each tooth is composed of the *crown*, which projects beyond the gum and is covered by *enamel*, the *neck* or cervical region, and the *root*, which is covered by *cement* and fixed into the alveolar bone of the maxilla or mandible by the fibrous *periodontal membrane* forming a *gomphosis*. The bulk of the tooth is formed of *dentine* which has the *pulp cavity* within it. This cavity is filled by the *pulp* which is a loose fibrous tissue contain-

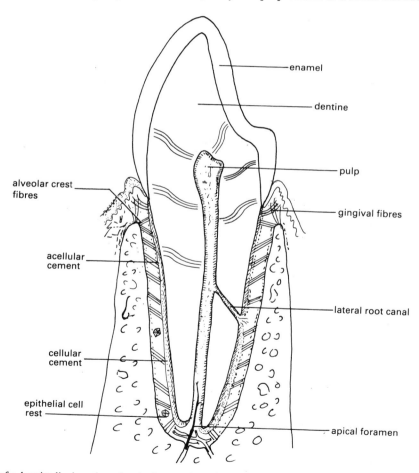

Fig. 1.1 Diagram of a longitudinal section of a single-rooted tooth.

ing nerves, blood vessels and lymphatics which pass into it via a foramen in the root apex.

Dentine and cement, both calcified, arise from mesoderm. Cement is like bone, with calcified lamellae. Dentine is harder, containing much organic material and also a system of spiral tubules which radiate outwards from the pulp cavity. Each contains a process of protoplasm from an *odontoblast* — one of the cells lining the pulp cavity. Odontoblasts have the capacity to produce dentine throughout life, depositing it on the inner surface of the dentine. Cement, too, can be produced throughout life; deposition, in this case, being on the outer surface.

Enamel, the third of the calcified tissues of the tooth, arises from epithelium and is the hardest tissue in the body. It is heavily calcified and non-vital and lacks the capacity to regenerate in response to injury.

The periodontal membrane consists of strong collagen fibres attached to the cement of the root. It is radiolucent. According to the direction in which these fibres run they can be divided into four groups:

1. Fibres passing from the cervical region of the teeth into the overlying gum. These *gingival* fibres hold the gum close to the neck of the teeth.

2. Fibres passing from the buccal and lingual cervical regions to the bone of the socket rim which resist tilting movements of the teeth. These are *alveolar crest* fibres.

3. Fibres which pass from the mesial and distal cervical region are
   a. *trans-septal* fibres and connect the necks of adjacent teeth and
   b. *cervical* fibres, which pass to the inner part of the sockets just below their rims.
These fibres hold the teeth together and resist tilting movements, respectively.

4. Fibres which form the bulk of the periodontal membrane and which run obliquely upwards from the cement of the root at one end to the alveolar bone at the other suspending the tooth firmly in its socket. These fibres transmit force from the tooth to the bone of the socket while allowing some degree of movement.

The normal width of the periodontal space is about 0.1–0.3 mm in functional teeth, being widest at the cervical and apical parts of the roots.

Deciduous dentition

The *deciduous* or milk teeth begin to appear at about the age of 6 months and are complete by about $2\frac{1}{2}$ years of age. They consist of 20 teeth when complete, 10 maxillary and 10 mandibular. There are 2 incisors, 1 canine and 2 deciduous molars in each half-jaw. In dental notation:

$$I_2^2 \; C_1^1 \; DM_2^2$$

The deciduous teeth are lost as the permanent teeth erupt. The deciduous molars precede the *premolar* teeth.

Permanent dentition

This first appears at about the 6th year of age, has replaced the deciduous dentition by the 13th year and is complete at or about the 20th year. There are 32 permanent teeth, half in the upper and half in the lower jaw. Two incisor, 1 canine, 2 premolar and 3 molar teeth are found in each half-jaw. The permanent molar teeth are not preceded by deciduous teeth and appear at the posterior parts of the dental arches as the jaws increase in size, i.e. at about the 6th, 12th and 18th years, respectively. In dental notation:

$$I_2^2 \; C_1^1 \; P_2^2 \; M_3^3$$

Times of eruption

Deciduous teeth

Lower central incisors	6 m
Upper central incisors	7 m
Lower lateral incisors	9 m
Upper lateral incisors	8 m
Canines	16–18 m
First molars	12–14 m
Second molars	2–$2\frac{1}{2}$ y
m = months postnatal,	y = years of age.

Permanent teeth

Central incisors	lower	6– 7 y
	upper	7– 8 y
Lateral incisors	lower	7– 8 y
	upper	8– 9 y
Canines	lower	9–10 y
	upper	11–12 y

First premolars	upper	10–11 y
	lower	10–12 y
Second premolars	upper	10–12 y
	lower	11–12 y
First permanent molars	upper	6– 7 y
	lower	6– 7 y
Second permanent molars	lower	11–13 y
	upper	12–13 y
Third permanent molars	upper	17–21 y
	lower	17–21 y

y = years of age

Tooth form

Teeth are shaped according to their function. Each has *mesial* (nearer the midline of the dental arch), *distal* (farther from the midline of the arch), *labial* (*buccal*) and *lingual* (*palatal*) surfaces. In premolar and molar teeth an *occlusal* surface is present. Each tooth, with the exception of the most distal teeth in each arch, is in contact with its neighbours.

Incisor teeth

As their name suggests, these teeth are shaped for cutting the food. The crowns of the incisors are chisel- or wedge-shaped, convex on their labial surfaces and concave on their lingual surfaces. In biting, the incisors first meet edge to edge and then the lower incisors slide up behind the upper ones in a 'slicing' action, like that of a pair of scissors.

Root form. The roots of the incisors are single and taper towards the apex. The upper roots are circular and the lower roots oval in cross-section; that of the lower central incisor may show some bifurcation.

Clinical considerations. The root apices of the upper incisors are close relations of the anterior part of the floor of the nose, those of the lower incisors lie above the genial tubercles.

In both upper and lower incisors the outer (labial) alveolar bone of their sockets is thinner than the inner (lingual) bone.

Supernumerary teeth are commonly found in the upper incisor region lying between or behind the normal teeth.

Upper lateral incisors are often deformed or absent. Crowding of lower incisors is common.

Canine teeth

The canine teeth lie behind the lateral incisors in the dental arch. They are prominent in the dog, from which their name derives, but do not project markedly in man. The crowns are more rugged than those of the incisors and are tipped by a pointed cusp. In lower canines this is not so obvious, the tooth being more like an incisor in shape. Canines are designed for gripping.

Root form. The roots of the canine teeth are normally single and conical. The lower canine may have two roots on occasion. Canine roots are stronger and longer than the roots of the other teeth.

Clinical considerations. The outer (labial) walls of the canine sockets are thinner than the inner (lingual) walls. The upper roots lie between the maxillary sinus and the lateral wall of the nose.

Premolar teeth

These teeth lie behind the canines and in front of the molar teeth in the dental arch. They replace the deciduous molar teeth but are completely different from them in crown and root form. They are used in crushing the food and have *occlusal* surfaces.

In premolar teeth the crowns are divided into two cusps, a *buccal* and a *lingual*, by a *fissure* running mesiodistally. In the first premolar teeth the buccal cusp is larger than the lingual whereas in the second premolars they are about the same size and the lingual cusp may be divided into two parts.

In the lower premolars the cusps are connected by a central ridge and the fissure separating them is therefore divided into two *fossae*, the distal being larger than the mesial. The ridge may be absent in the lower second premolar.

Root form. The upper first premolar usually possesses two roots — a buccal and a lingual root — although the point at which they bifurcate may vary considerably. Sometimes this tooth may have a single root and, rarely, three roots — two buccal and one lingual. The upper second premolar has a single root, occasionally double.

The lower premolars have single roots often curving in a distal direction to the apex, that of the lower first premolar may be bifurcated close to the apex.

Clinical considerations. The outer (buccal) walls of the sockets of the premolars are thinner than the inner walls. The root apex of the upper second premolar is related to the maxillary sinus, the apices of the lower premolars lie above the mylohyoid line.

Molar teeth

These teeth lie behind the premolars in the dental arch and are designed for grinding and crushing food between their occlusal surfaces.

Of the upper molars the first molar is the largest and its crown possesses four cusps called, according to their position, *mesiobuccal, mesiolingual, distobuccal* and *distolingual* cusps. The largest cusp, the mesiolingual, is joined to the distobuccal cusp by a ridge which divides the occlusal surface of the tooth into mesial and distal fossae, the former being the larger.

In over half of these teeth a fifth cusp — the tubercle of Carabelli — is found on the lingual side of the mesiolingual cusp.

The upper second molar is similar but smaller than the first. It also has four cusps, the distolingual and distobuccal being smaller in size and the former may be absent.

The upper third molar is smaller than the upper second and is frequently tricuspid, the distolingual cusp being absent.

The lower first molar tooth has five cusps. Four, like the cusps of the upper molars, are named in the same fashion, the mesial pair being larger than the distal pair; the fifth is called the *distal* cusp and is placed distally between the distobuccal and distolingual cusps. A sixth, *paramolar*, cusp is rarely present on the buccal surface. The crown of this tooth has a central fossa and the cusps are separated from each other by fissures radiating out from it.

The lower second molar is similar to the lower first, though smaller, and the distal cusp is usually absent leaving a cruciate fissure pattern.

The lower third molar may be larger or smaller than the lower second and has four or five cusps which are subject to considerable variation.

Root form. The upper molars have three roots each. They arise from a common undivided portion below the necks of the teeth and are named the *mesiobuccal, distobuccal* and *palatal* (lingual) roots from their respective positions. In terms of length and strength the palatal root is pre-eminent, then the mesiobuccal and finally the distobuccal root. The palatal root diverges from the other two roots in the first upper molar but is less divergent in the second upper molar and may even unite with one of the buccal roots. In the third upper molar all the roots are often fused into a single mass.

The lower molar teeth have two roots each — a *mesial* and a *distal* — again arising from a common undivided part below the neck of the tooth. The mesial is larger than the distal root. In the lower first molar the apex of the mesial root curves distally, that of the distal root may also curve slightly in the same direction. In the lower second and third molars both roots curve distally. Occasionally the roots of the lower second molar are fused. The third molar roots are smaller than those of the second and are often fused.

Clinical considerations. The outer (buccal) walls of the upper molar sockets are thinner than the inner (palatal) walls and the roots of the teeth are closely related to the floor of the maxillary sinus.

The outer walls of the lower third molar sockets are very thick and become progressively thinner in the sockets of the lower second and lower first molars. Below the mylohyoid line lie the root apices of the third and occasionally the second molar.

Tooth development (Fig. 1.2)

Prior to the development of the teeth, the primitive mouth (stomatodeum) is lined by columnar epithelium. At about the fourth embryonic week a localised proliferation of the basal layer of this epithelium forms an arc-like structure which overlies each jaw and projects into the underlying mesoderm. It is believed that this proliferation may be induced by cells of neural crest origin (ectomesenchyme cells) which have migrated into this area.

This proliferation forms the *primary epithelial band* or the *odontogenic epithelium* which, in the fifth week, is seen to occupy six separate zones

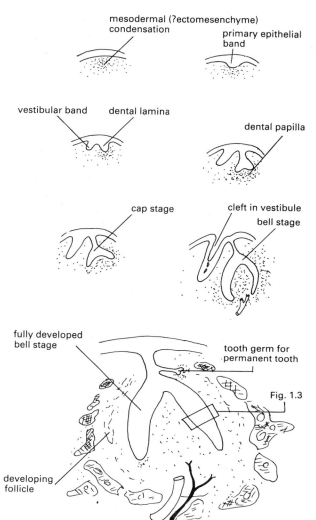

Fig. 1.2 The stages in the development of a tooth up to the late bell stage.

deep surface of the now shelf-like dental lamina, at about the eighth week, small buds grow and penetrate the surrounding mesenchyme to form, initially, the *enamel organs* of the deciduous teeth and, much later, those for the permanent molars.

The mesoderm in relation to each bud proliferates to form a dense mass of cells, the *dental papilla*. The deep surface of the bud invaginates soon after to form the *cap stage* of the enamel organ and as this grows and deepens it gradually encloses the dental papilla within it. With growth the cap of the enamel organ deepens further into a bell-shape — the *bell stage* of development — almost completely surrounding the dental papilla. At about this time a cleft appears in the vestibular band which will eventually separate the lips and cheeks from the gums.

The dental lamina continues to grow backwards in both jaws from the area of the deciduous tooth germs. It is in this posterior area that the enamel organs of the permanent molars appear and grow in the same way as those of the deciduous teeth, but much later in time.

The cells forming the inner (within the bell) and the outer layers of the enamel organ differ. The cells of the outer layer are low columnar cells and form the *external enamel epithelium*, those of the inner layer are taller and form the *internal enamel epithelium*. The cells of the enamel organ which lie between these two layers are more rounded and although tightly packed in the cap stage have, by the bell stage, separated into a loosely packed and delicate *stellate reticulum*.

By the late bell stage a fourth cell layer is visible. It is two to three cells deep, lies between the inner enamel epithelium and the stellate reticulum, and is known as the *stratum intermedium*.

Continued growth of the enamel organ occurs throughout fetal life at the 'rim' of the bell, i.e. where the internal and external enamel epithelia are continuous — an area known as the *cervical loop* of the organ.

As the cells of the enamel organ grow and differentiate into their four layers changes also appear in the dental papilla. Capillaries form to nourish the tissue and simple nerve fibres enter it. A marked increase in the innervation of the papilla is evident soon after birth.

As the tooth develops, an aggregation of meso-

— an area on each mandibular arch which will extend to the midline and fuse, an area on each lateral border of the frontonasal process, and an area on each maxillary process. The latter four zones fuse into one plate soon afterwards. In the seventh week the primary epithelial band divides into two processes; the *vestibular band* placed buccally, which first marks off and later divides the lips and cheeks from the gums, and the *dental lamina* placed lingually, which will give rise to the ectodermal parts of the teeth.

With proliferation the dental lamina gradually penetrates into the deeper tissues and from the

dermal cells lies in contact with the external enamel epithelium and encloses it and the dental papilla within a sac. It develops into the *dental follicle* which is a nutritive capsule around the tooth. The follicle finally forms the periodontal membrane of the tooth.

Once the enamel organ has enclosed the area of the developing tooth crown it continues to grow and produce the root area. In this area the internal and external enamel epithelia grow as a two-layered epithelium, not separated by the stratum intermedium and the stellate reticulum, known as the *sheath of Hertwig*. Growth of this sheath forms the roots of the tooth in the same way as the enamel organ forms the crown, by enclosing the dental papilla. In the formation of a single root the sheath is tubular but in the formation of two or more roots this simple tube is subdivided by extensions of the epithelium inwards to form as many tubes as there will be roots.

Once differentiation of enamel organ cells occurs the formation of dentine and enamel begins, commencing at the cusps of the grinding teeth and the incisive edges of the cutting teeth even before the full area of the crown has been demarcated by the growing enamel organ.

Soon after the start of dentine and enamel formation in the enamel organs of the deciduous teeth the dental lamina begins to degenerate, breaking up into clumps of epithelial cells around the developing teeth. Also about this time the enamel organs for the *successional permanent teeth* (those with deciduous predecessors) begin to form on the lingual side of the deciduous enamel organs already present. They arise in the same way and pass through the same stages of growth as the deciduous enamel organs.

The developing tooth, within its follicle, begins to form an attachment with the alveolar bone once root formation begins. Prior to that the follicle has lain independently within a trough of bone which is subsequently subdivided into alveoli for each tooth. As the tooth grows resorption of the alveolar bone occurs to make room for it. The mucous membrane of the gums thickens over the alveoli forming *gum pads*.

The successional permanent teeth lie lingually in the same follicles as their predecessors until these erupt and then gain their own follicles, attached to the oral mucous membrane by fibrous *gubernacular cords*. The now separate follicles lodge in the alveolar bone in separate cavities or *crypts* which are open above to allow passage of the gubernacular cords which either lie lingual to the erupted deciduous teeth or within the sockets of their predecessors (as is the case with the premolar teeth).

Dentine formation (Fig. 1.3)

The cells of the dental papilla are mesodermal in origin and are separated from the cells of the internal enamel epithelium by a basement membrane. Those cells of the dental papilla which lie adjacent to this membrane differentiate, under the influence of the internal enamel epithelium, into *odontoblasts* which produce *predentine*. Predentine is deposited adjacent to the basement membrane which then forms the enamel-dentine junction.

After a time, calcification of the predentine forms true dentine, occurring first in the older predentine and following predentine formation as the odontoblasts retreat inwards into the dental papilla leaving protoplasmic processes behind them, each in its own spiral tubule. The thickness of the dentine formed depends on the distance the odontoblasts migrate in any given area and, as the dentine thickens, so is the size of the pulp cavity reduced.

Dentine is laid down in a periodic fashion and this results in *incremental lines* in the dentine. *Peritubular* dentine, varying slightly in composition from the rest of the dentine, is laid down within each spiral tubule. The dentine of the root area is laid down later, during eruption of the tooth, in the same manner as the coronal dentine but under the influence of the sheath of Hertwig, not the internal enamel epithelium.

The dentine of the crown and root that is thus formed is the *primary dentine* but formation of dentine can occur throughout life and this normal or physiological *secondary dentine* is deposited on the inner surface of the primary dentine and so gradually reduces the size of the pulp cavity. Secondary dentine is of two types: *regular* secondary dentine, which is formed in response to mild damage of the primary dentine and which is similar to primary

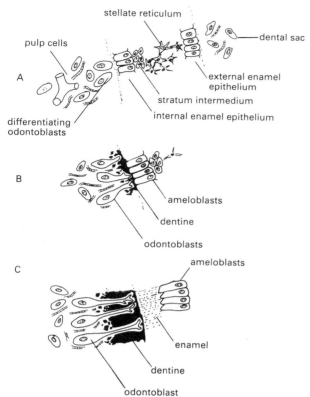

Fig. 1.3 Diagrams showing the formation of enamel and dentine. A — A high power view of the boxed area indicated in the late bell stage in Figure 1.2. The different cell types in the enamel organ are shown. B — Early dentinogenesis. C — Diagram showing the formation of enamel & dentinal tubules.

dentine in the arrangement of the tubules; and *irregular* secondary dentine, formed in response to stronger stimuli and in which the tubules are arranged less regularly and may be absent altogether.

Regular secondary dentine is usually laid down over the whole internal surface of the primary dentine, irregular secondary dentine is usually formed in localised areas related to the damaged areas of primary dentine.

Stimuli applied to dentine by attrition or caries formation also results in areas of *translucent* dentine or *dead tracts*. In the former the tubules become gradually blocked by calcified material and appear lucent under transmitted light and in the latter the affected odontoblasts and their processes die, the tubules are blocked by secondary dentine deposits and they appear opaque under transmitted light.

Enamel formation (Fig. 1.3)

Soon after the start of formation of dentine by the odontoblasts the cells of the internal enamel epithelium of the crown differentiate to form *ameloblasts* which produce enamel. The basement membrane separating these cells from the odontoblasts disappears.

Initially, enamel is deposited at the *enamel-dentine junction* in the areas of the cusps or incisive edges, depending on the type of teeth involved. The initial deposition is of a highly organic enamel matrix secreted through the *Tomes processes* of the ameloblasts. (Tomes processes are pyramidal extensions of cytoplasm at the formative end of the cells.) Soon after matrix deposition crystals of hydroxy-apatite are deposited in the matrix in a prism pattern, the direction of which is related to one of the surfaces of the Tomes process. Migration of ameloblasts away from the site of enamel deposition also occurs in this direction.

Retreat of the ameloblast layer is accompanied by loss of the stellate reticulum, which brings the ameloblasts and the stratum intermedium into close contact with the dental follicle and its capillaries. The stratum intermedium then disappears as the enamel becomes mature, leaving the surface enamel covered by the ameloblast layer (now indistinguishable from the external enamel epithelium) and the remains of the enamel organ, a structure known as the reduced enamel epithelium, continuous below with the sheath of Hertwig. This covering protects the enamel from the tissues of the follicle before eruption and provides an epithelial pathway for the tooth during eruption by fusing with the oral epithelium.

The enamel prisms are arranged roughly perpendicularly to the surface of the dentine. Their course is not straight but wavy, especially at the cusps where it is stronger and is known as *gnarled enamel*. These alterations of direction of the prisms also give rise to an optical phenomenon known as *Hunter-Schreger lines*, under oblique light.

Enamel, like dentine, is laid down in bursts which give rise to *incremental lines* (brown striae of Retzius) representing the enamel in its stages of formation.

The inner enamel surface where it is attached

to the dentine has a 'scalloped' appearance which strengthens the junction between the two materials.

Cement formation (Fig. 1.4)

The dentine of the root is, at first, covered by the sheath of Hertwig and, when it disintegrates, the dentine comes into contact with cells of the follicle which differentiate into *cementoblasts*. Cement matrix is first laid down on the dentine and subsequently calcified. Fibres from the periodontal membrane are imbedded into the cement.

Cement is very similar to bone and is of two types — *acellular* and *cellular*. Acellular cement is formed first, lacks cells within it and coats the whole root in a thin layer from the enamel-cement junction to near the root apex. Cellular cement is formed secondarily, contains cells (cementocytes) distributed irregularly in lacunae throughout it and is found mainly at the root apices. It may be thin or absent in incisor and canine teeth and appears at the time of tooth eruption.

In the majority of people the cement overlaps the enamel at the enamel-cement junction but may meet it edge to edge or not at all; in the latter case leaving dentine exposed. The junction of cement and enamel is often exposed as the gums migrate rootwards with age.

Pulp

The remnants of the dental papilla following dentine formation form the *pulp*. It is located in the *pulp cavity* of the teeth and is composed of loose connective tissue and cells, with vascular, neural and lymphatic elements passing into and out of it via the *root foramina* of the root apices.

The pulp cavity is composed of the *pulp chamber* which occupies the crown of the tooth, *cornua* or *horns* which project cuspally from the pulp chamber and *pulp canals* which are located in the roots of the teeth and which may vary considerably in form and number.

The blood vessels and nerves of the pulp are nutritive and sensory to the surrounding dentine, respectively. The reaction of the pulp to stimuli, of whatever cause, is *pain* with the production of

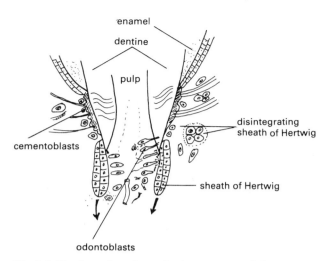

Fig. 1.4 The formation of root dentine, cement and the sheath of Hertwig. Cellular remnants of the sheath of Hertwig may persist in the periodontal membrane.

secondary dentine by the odontoblast layer on the surface of the pulp or, in severe cases, inflammation of the pulp.

Odontoblasts form the outer layer of the pulp. Beneath them is the *basal layer of Weil*, a zone with few cells, and, below that, the other cells, fibres and vessels of the pulp. This area of the pulp is composed of a gelatinous ground substance bound together by fine collagenous fibres in which lie numerous fibroblasts, macrophages, lymphocytes and undifferentiated mesenchyme cells.

Located within the pulp are numerous blood vessels which consist of arterioles passing into the pulp through the apical foramina which then branch and anastomose with each other forming a rich vascular plexus. These vessels drain into large venules which exit through the same foramina together with lymphatic vessels.

Nerve fibres enter through the apical foramina in close association with the blood vessels and branch to form a rich plexus (plexus of Raschkow) below the cell-sparse zone of Weil. Fibres from this plexus pass to the odontoblast layer and the predentine; most then pass back towards the pulp but some branches can be traced into the dentinal tubules. These nerve fibres are of the somatic sensory group carrying pain sensation only but some autonomic fibres are also present and supply the blood vessels.

Eruption

This term covers not only the *emergence* of the tooth into the oral cavity but the continuous movement involved in carrying the tooth from the alveolus or crypt through the gum into the mouth and finally into occlusion.

The exact cause of eruption is not known but many theories have been put forward in explanation. For instance:

1. *Root growth*: this postulates that the growing root thrusts the crown into the mouth and has been shown to be unlikely by (a) experiment on rodent incisors where the incisal and basal parts of the tooth have been separated and yet the incisal part erupts like an intact tooth and (b) the fact that teeth with *no roots* — 'neonatal' teeth — or teeth with *fully formed* roots may erupt.

2. *Pulp growth*: as with root growth the mechanism suggested is similar; that eruption takes place by pulpal proliferation pushing the crown outwards. Administration of substances which prevent mitosis does reduce eruption but whether this is due to the decrease in *pulpal* mitoses is not known, since mitosis in other cells is also prevented. It may be that root and pulp growth takes place as a *result* of eruption, simply to fill the space left behind by the moving tooth.

3. *Tissue fluid pressure*: as in 1. and 2. above, the motive force is here thought to be an increase in tissue fluid or blood pressure at the apical region of the erupting tooth. Pressure differentials have been found by experiment on dogs.

4. *Bone growth*: selective resorption and deposition of bone beneath the erupting tooth may provide the necessary force. Studies have shown that deposition of bone 'fills-in' the space left *after* the tooth has moved.

5. *Periodontal fibres*: unlike 1. to 4. above, this postulates a *pulling* force acting on the erupting tooth. This theory is tenable since (a) contraction occurs in developing collagen fibres which may be aided by shrinkage of fibres by dehydration; (b) if synthesis of collagen is experimentally disturbed eruption is slowed although root growth continues, and (c) since root growth seems to bear no part in eruption [see 1(a) above] then the decrease in eruption produced by substances which prevent

mitosis may be caused by their action on cells in the periodontal ligament.

Notwithstanding, the cause of eruption is still unclear but it is probable that it is multifactorial.

Eruption is a continuous process which begins upon completion of formation of the crown after which it begins to move upwards towards its final position in the mouth. Proliferation of the sheath of Hertwig follows, initiating the formation of the root which is constantly growing during crown movement and at emergence of the tooth is about three-quarters formed.

In deciduous teeth the crown moves through the overlying gum, which becomes looser due to increased vascularity and the presence within it of cysts from the disintegrating dental lamina. In permanent teeth, enclosed almost totally within their crypts, the roof of the crypt resorbs, the gubernacular canal enlarges and the cord becomes more vascular and looser, and the tooth erupts along its line.

The enamel of the crown is covered and protected by the reduced enamel epithelium, continuous below with the sheath of Hertwig. As the crown reaches the oral epithelium the reduced enamel epithelium fuses with it and the tooth erupts bloodlessly through this area. The crown is now only partially covered by the reduced enamel epithelium which forms the boundary between the tooth and the gum. With more growth this boundary retreats towards the cervical area of the tooth with consequent exposure of more of the crown. *Active eruption*, with movement of the tooth relative to the surrounding tissues, ceases when the tooth is in occlusion but this uncovering of the crown — *passive eruption* — continues until not only the crown but some of the root is exposed.

During eruption the dental follicle differentiates to form the periodontal membrane and the alveolus or crypt forms the close-fitting tooth socket.

Deciduous teeth

The deciduous teeth start to appear in the mouth at about 6 months of age and are complete by the age of 2 to $2\frac{1}{2}$ years. They appear at intervals and usually in the following order:

$I_1 \; I_2 \; DM_1 \; C \; DM_2$

Formation of their roots is complete 1 to $1\frac{1}{2}$ years after the tooth appears.

Permanent teeth

As the deciduous teeth erupt the crowns of their permanent successors are forming. They subsequently erupt after a period of quiescence and this initiates the formation of their roots.

The permanent teeth first appear at about the age of 6 years and are complete by about the age of 21 years. They usually erupt in the following order:

$(M_1 I_1) I_2 (C P_1 P_2 M_2) M_3,$

but variation does occur. Lower incisor teeth usually erupt before upper incisors.

Shedding of deciduous teeth

Each deciduous tooth is replaced by a permanent tooth. The permanent molars have no deciduous predecessors. The process of removal of deciduous teeth is known as *shedding* and occurs earlier in the female.

The permanent teeth lie separate from the deciduous teeth within crypts which are connected to the oral cavity by the gubernacular cords. As they erupt they exert pressure on the adjacent tissues and this leads to resorption, first of the bone of the crypt and then of the cement and dentine of the deciduous root. Resorption proceeds crownwards as the permanent tooth continues to erupt.

Permanent incisors and canine teeth initially lie deep and lingual to the roots of their deciduous predecessors. Resorption, therefore, first affects the lingual side of the root apices. Later these permanent teeth come to lie more directly under the deciduous teeth and resorption affects the whole of the root. The premolar teeth are situated deep to their predecessors and resorption affects these root apices first.

Resorption occurs in bouts with a certain amount of repair occurring in between and continues until all or almost all of the root is gone, whereupon the tooth is shed and replaced by a permanent tooth.

Shedding of deciduous teeth is brought about by root resorption aided by an increase in growth and masticatory load with ageing for which the deciduous roots are inadequate.

Clinical considerations of tooth development

A. During the development of the teeth many variations from the normal may occur in the form, number and size of the teeth.

Tooth form

1. Variations in the overall form of the teeth may range from minor abnormalities to gross deformities. Teeth may have more or less than their normal complement of cusps. The number of roots may exceed the norm or they may be fused together. The distortion may be so great that the tooth bears no resemblance to its normal counterpart.

2. The various dental epithelia may not develop normally resulting in abnormal and irregular arrangements of the tissues of the tooth. These arrangements may be cellular, e.g. ameloblastomata, or form masses of calcified tissues either single — complex composite odontome — or multiple — compound composite odontomes.

Abnormal forms of teeth are more frequently found in cases of mental retardation.

Tooth number

More or less teeth than the normal complement may be found.

1. *Supernumerary teeth* — an excess in the normal number of teeth is uncommon in the deciduous dentition but may be caused in the permanent dentition by, it is thought:
   a. extra deciduous or permanent enamel organs,
   b. splitting of an enamel organ, or
   c. budding-off of a lamina from a permanent enamel organ.

In the condition known as cleidocranial dysostosis many extra teeth are found and usually remain unerupted. More commonly, one or more supernumerary teeth may be found in the incisor or molar areas. This occurs in 1–3% of people, and is more common in males.

2. *Oligodontia* (hypodontia) — less than the nor-

mal number of teeth due to a decreased number of enamel organs. In extreme forms there may be no teeth at all (anodontia). Oligodontia is common in the permanent dentition. The third molar is most affected followed by the second premolars and upper lateral incisors.

Tooth size

Variations in size may affect the root or crown only or the whole tooth. There is normally some variation in the size of teeth but unusually large or small teeth may be found.

B. Following the disintegration of the dental lamina remnants of it may lie between the developing crowns and the overlying oral epithelium. Some of these may proliferate to form small epithelial masses — the *glands of Serres* — and may proceed to form cysts.

Enamel

1. Developmental disturbances may affect formation or calcification of the matrix.

   a. *Matrix formation*: if disturbed, leads to enamel *hypoplasia* which may appear as a localised single defect, multiple defects or affect the whole enamel. Such defects appearing in one permanent tooth may be caused by sepsis in its deciduous predecessor but these defects are frequently seen in a number of teeth and affect the enamel matrix that was being produced at the time of the causative insult, e.g. hypoparathyroidism, vitamin D deficiency. The enamel of all the teeth may be affected in a hereditary condition known as *amelogenesis imperfecta*.

   b. *Calcification*: if disturbed, produces enamel *hypocalcification*, the main cause being excessive fluorine levels in drinking water leading to the condition known as 'mottled enamel'.

2. Enamel is very hard but is brittle and liable to fracture if unsupported therefore care must be taken in cavity preparation.

Dentine

1. Dental caries nearly always produces dead tracts through the underlying dentine. These run in the direction of the affected dentinal tubules and are sealed at their pulpal ends by formation of irregular secondary dentine thereby preventing the spread of decay into the pulp. If, in cavity preparation, only this sealed dead tract is cut into but no unsealed tubules are opened then no exposure of the pulp will occur.

2. Formation of regular secondary dentine decreases the size of the pulp cavity but by the same token also decreases the likelihood of pulp exposure by attrition or cavity preparation.

3. With age, much of the dentine, especially of the roots, becomes translucent.

Pulp

1. The pulp cavity of teeth is gradually reduced by deposition of regular secondary dentine with age. In parts, especially the floor of the pulp chamber of multirooted teeth, this deposition is very thick. Deposition of irregular secondary dentine also reduces the pulp cavity but in an irregular fashion.

2. Root canals may be single, double or multiple and variations of all these may occur at different places in the same root. The canal may be naturally irregular or become irregular through localised deposits of irregular secondary dentine.

3. Apical foramina are frequently not single, there may be two or three foramina and they may be located not at the apex but to the side of it.

4. *Lateral root canals* may be present anywhere along the length of the root canal.

5. With age, the odontoblasts lining the pulp cavity degenerate, the fibre content of the pulp increases and the number of cells, nerve bundles and blood vessels decreases. This results in a decreased response to stimulation. Deposits of calcium, either localised — *pulp stones* — or diffuse, also appear.

6. The opening up of healthy dentinal tubules exposes the pulp and produces a reaction. If this is mild it leads to the formation of secondary dentine, if severe to inflammation of the pulp — *pulpitis*. This response on the part of the pulp may be caused during cavity or crown preparation by unnecessary damage due to the excessive production of heat by drilling, by the opening up of undamaged dentinal tubules (those not sealed pul-

pally by secondary dentine) or by the use of irritant filling materials.

Inflammation of the pulp leads to an increase of pressure within the pulp cavity and consequent pain. Blood vessels, especially within the narrow foramina, may be occluded by this pressure.

Cement

1. Occasionally a part of the sheath of Hertwig develops to form a small area of enamel organ. This leads to the formation of an *enamel pearl* within the surrounding cement.

2. Imbedded within the cement are the fibres of the periodontal membrane. These are not, however, static and with movement of the tooth either vertically in eruption or laterally and mesially during growth and attrition the place of attachment of the fibres alters according to the positional or functional alteration undergone by the affected tooth. This principle is of vital importance in orthodontic dentistry since pressure can be applied to a tooth to move it artificially into a new and more desirable functional or cosmetic position. These pressures need to be low, however, since damage, excessive resorption or necrosis of the cement may occur if excessive pressures are used.

3. Ossification between the tooth and its socket is usually prevented by the movement between them but may occur, usually in retained deciduous teeth where loading forces are taken by adjacent permanent teeth and movement is diminished. Ossification or *ankylosis* may also occur with chronic inflammation in permanent teeth.

4. *Hypercementosis*: chronic inflammation around the roots commonly gives rise to the deposition of cement with a marked increase in root thickness which may affect the whole root or the apex only. Hypercementosis may affect one or more teeth and make the extraction of such teeth difficult.

5. With gingival recession cement may become exposed. Exposed cement loses its vitality with loss of nutrition from the gum and the periodontal membrane and may be worn away by attrition or during careless scaling.

Periodontal membrane

1. The tissues of the dental follicle which will form the future periodontal membrane come into contact with the developing cement upon disintegration of the sheath of Hertwig. Remnants of the sheath, known as *epithelial debris*, may be found particularly at root apices and may proliferate, especially in the presence of chronic inflammation, to form cysts.

2. Since the periodontal membrane is attached both to the cement and to the alveolar bone of the socket, if excessive or misplaced force is used in extraction of a tooth parts of the alveolar bone may fracture and be removed adhering to the tooth.

3. Infections of the pulp may spread through the apical foramen to involve the periodontal membrane producing an *apical abscess*. This may spread into the adjacent bone or open into the floor of the mouth or nasal cavity, the pterygopalatine fossa or the maxillary sinus depending on its situation. With age the bone of the upper molar sockets may become resorbed allowing an easier spread of infection into the maxillary sinus.

The periodontal membrane may be infected from the oral cavity by a descending infection of the gum (gingivitis) which may also affect the alveolar bone resulting in a loose tooth.

Eruption

1. Deciduous teeth may remain in position beyond the time at which they are normally shed. This may be due to:

  a The crown remaining in position after the roots have been resorbed due to the attachment of its pulp to the surrounding tissues and also because of the attachment of the gingival tissues to the crown.

  b. Non-formation of the replacing permanent tooth. This occurs most frequently in the lower second premolar, and also affects the upper lateral incisor.

  c. Failure of the permanent replacement to erupt. Frequently affects upper canine teeth.

  d. Overactive repair of the deciduous roots during a quiescent phase of resorption. This may lead to *ankylosis* of the deciduous tooth in which the cement and the alveolar bone become united.

In b. and c. above, the deciduous tooth will eventually be shed by root resorption caused by an increased masticatory load. In d. above, the ankylosed tooth may prevent eruption of the permanent tooth or cause it to erupt into an abnormal position. The trapped deciduous tooth may fail to rise with the increase in height of the alveolar bone during growth and may gradually come to lie in a much lower position relative to adjacent teeth. This may take place to such an extent that the tooth becomes buried in the alveolar bone.

2. Fragments of the deciduous roots may be unresorbed and left in the tissues during shedding. This occurs most frequently in the deciduous second molars, the fragments remaining between the roots of the erupted permanent teeth.

3. *Cysts*: some cysts arising from the remains of the dental lamina may become quite large. Occasionally they lie between the tooth and the overlying gum and are known as *cysts of eruption*. These usually disappear on emergence of the tooth but may envelop the crown forming a *dentigerous cyst*.

4. Beneath the oral epithelium is an aggregation of mesoderm with which the tooth germs or follicles are kept in developmental contact. Should this connection be lost the tooth may become deeply imbedded within the jaw or erupt in an abnormal position, for example, into the nasal cavity, pterygopalatine fossa or beneath the chin. This situation is more likely in the permanent dentition due to rupture of the gubernacular cord and may follow on from a fractured jaw or by scar formation round a follicle after infection.

5. Eruption of the deciduous teeth is delayed in 'small for dates' babies and in those suffering from severe malnutrition.

6. A form of active eruption can occur later in life due to attrition. Eruption of the teeth occurs as they are worn down so as to maintain them in occlusion.

7. The *anatomical crown* refers to that part of the tooth which is covered by the enamel. The *clinical crown* is that part of the tooth which is exposed in the mouth. The clinical crown is at first smaller than the anatomical crown but with the movement of the gum tissues cervically during eruption they become the same size and later, with partial exposure of the root, the clinical crown exceeds the anatomical crown in size.

In primitive races the process of passive eruption (uncovering of the crown) keeps pace with attrition of the teeth and the active eruption which goes with it. Passive eruption in this case may thus be considered a normal or physiological phenomenon. In more civilised man marked attrition is lost and passive eruption leads to the appearance of very long clinical crowns in which case it may be considered as abnormal. Passive eruption is accelerated in gingivitis.

GINGIVAL TISSUES (Fig. 1.5)

The gingivae are composed of dense vascular fibrous tissue covered with keratinised stratified squamous epithelium. They consist of two parts: the *free gingiva*, which surrounds the neck of the tooth like a snug collar, and the *attached gingiva*, which is anchored to the periosteum of the alveolar bone.

The gingiva is pale pink in colour, firm to the touch and relatively insensitive to moderate pressure. It has a finely stippled 'orange peel' surface. In children the gingivae are redder in colour and lack the surface stippling seen in the adult.

The attached gingivae are continuous at the lingual, labial and buccal sulci with the mucosa of the floor of the mouth, lips and cheeks respectively. This is redder in colour, glossy and unstippled. The attached gingiva related to the palatal aspect of the maxillary teeth is continuous with the mucoperiosteum of the palate.

The free gingiva is closely applied to the neck of a tooth (Fig. 1.5). The epithelial component of the gingiva in contact with the tooth is called the *epithelial attachment* and is derived from a fusion of oral epithelium and reduced enamel epithelium. The epithelial attachment is continuous with the epithelium of the *gingival crevice*. It is a nonkeratinised stratified squamous epithelium whose surface is in contact with the tooth.

The enamel surface related to the gingiva is covered by an *enamel cuticle*. The cells of the epithelial attachment are intimately and perhaps organically attached to the enamel cuticle forming a living functional barrier to the invasion of irritants and micro-organisms into the underlying connective tissue.

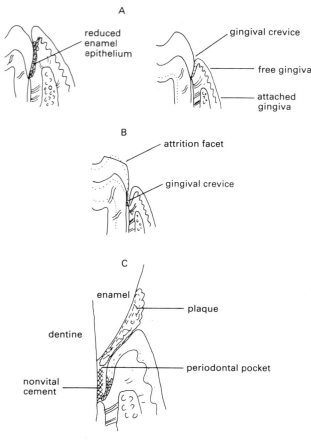

Fig. 1.5 A — The epithelial attachment forms during the last stages of eruption as the reduced enamel epithelium fuses with the oral epithelium. B — Passive eruption causes the epithelium to pass onto the tooth root. C — Diagram showing how plaque can disrupt the normal anatomical arrangement of the gingival tissues.

Clinical considerations

Dental plaque is a thin film of material which is deposited on the exposed surfaces of teeth. It is composed of micro-organisms of the oral flora and amorphous oral debris. Plaque can be removed readily, e.g. by tooth brushing, but reforms within a few hours. Deposits of plaque will accumulate in areas which are not amenable to effective removal, such as interstitial regions and the occlusal pits and fissures.

Stains. Stained deposits may also accumulate on tooth surfaces. The materials involved vary from tobacco tars and residues to salivary muco- and glyco-proteins. The acquired films may have dif-ferent colours. Tobacco staining is a brown to black colour. In other stains, chromogenic organisms give colours which vary from black to green.

Calculus. In many individuals, hard mineral deposits gather on the teeth. The deposits usually occur at specific sites related to the openings of the salivary gland ducts. The lingual surfaces of the lower anterior teeth and the buccal surfaces of the maxillary molars are the common sites of deposition. Calculus formation requires the deposition of an organic matrix similar to plaque onto the tooth surface. Mineralisation of the matrix then occurs and inorganic phosphates, principally calcium, are laid down forming the characteristic concreted deposit. Calculus can gather *supragingivally* and *subgingivally* relative to the lip of the gingival crevice. Since its presence distorts the normal anatomy and function of the gingival tissues and contains microorganisms it may produce an associated gingivitis.

Diseases of dental tissues (Table 1.1)

1. *Dental caries* is the most prevalent chronic disease that affects humans. It is characterised by the *demineralisation* of the calcified components and the *destruction* of the organic portions of teeth. Its initiation is dependent on the presence of microorganisms in dental plaque on the enamel surface and hence is more liable to occur at those sites where the attempted removal of plaque is inadequate.

Progressive decalcification of enamel and dentine allows micro-organisms to proliferate in the by now soft tooth substance. Further invasion of micro-organisms has a deleterious effect on the pulp and *pulpitis* occurs. If untreated, the microorganisms can gain access to the dental pulp and this results in an open pulpitis in which the pulp communicates with the oral cavity. Spread of the infection through the root canals occurs and the apical periodontal tissues become infected.

2. *Inflammatory disease of periodontal tissues.* Inflammatory conditions of the gingival tissue, *gingivitis*, and of the periodontal tissues, *periodontitis*, are common. Gingivitis occurs in *acute* or *chronic* forms. Among the many local and systemic factors involved are the presence of dental plaque or calculus and malposition of teeth. In most cases, no specific micro-organism is involved. Untreated

Table 1.1 Diseases of dental tissues

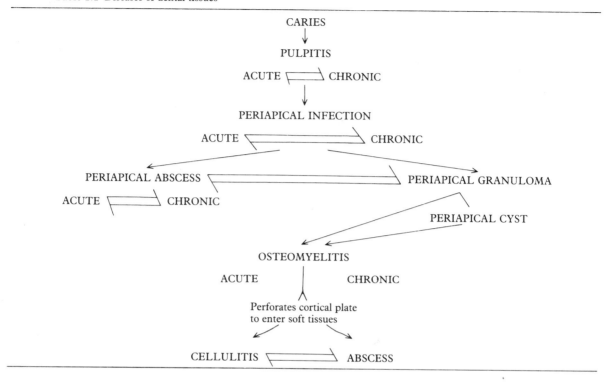

gingivitis can progress as the integrity of the gingival epithelium is lost to involve the deeper periodontal tissues causing a periodontitis. The classic lesion is the *periodontal pocket*. Destruction of the periodontal attachment involving alveolar bone resorption takes place and the teeth become mobile.

Acute ulcerative gingivitis is an infection of the gingiva caused by specific micro-organisms, fusiform bacilli and *Borrelia vincenti* acting symbiotically. It is characterised by ulceration and destruction of the interdental papilla. It can be treated successfully with cleansing procedures and/or antibiotics. If destruction of the interdental papilla has been marked, the restoration of the gingival contours during healing may be abnormal and predispose to gingivitis and gingival recession.

Gingival hyperplasia can occur in inflammatory and noninflammatory types. The hyperplasia may occur *focally* or be *generalised*. Inflammatory hyperplasia is frequently seen in chronic gingivitis or in endocrine disturbances such as occur in puberty or pregnancy. More seriously, gingival hyperplasia can occur in leukaemia when the gingival tissues become engorged with abnormal leukocytes. Noninflammatory hyperplasia presents as a focal hyperplasia of the fibrous tissue in one or more interdental papillae. Fibrous hyperplasia of the gingiva occurs frequently in patients treated with the anticonvulsant drug diphenylhydantoin. This may be so severe as to interfere with function and surgical excision may be necessary. However, the hyperplasia recurs under the influence of the drug.

Spread of infections of dental origin (Fig. 1.6)

Pulpal or superficial periodontal infections spread to involve the periapical tissues. The infection will show a tendency to *spread through* or remain *localised* in the cancellous bone. This is determined by the nature of the micro-organism and the defence response of the tissues.

Periapical infections are acute or chronic. Suppurative infections lead to the formation of a *dental abscess*. In chronic periapical infections the characteristic lesion is the *periapical granuloma*. In this the infective inflammatory process is accompanied by granuloma formation indicating a reparative process. As the granulation tissues proliferate, the surrounding bone is placed under pressure and is *resorbed*. The presence of bone resorption is evident radiographically as an *area of radiolucency* related to the root apex.

Periapical cysts

The presence of epithelial remnants of tooth formation (cell rests of Malassez) commonly results in the development of cysts in chronic periapical granulomata. The inflammatory process in the granuloma stimulates the epithelial cells to proliferate forming a cystic cavity lined by stratified squamous epithelium enclosed in a condensed fibrous tissue wall. The lumen of the cyst is fluid filled. *Osteomyelitis* of the alveolar bone can result from periapical infections particularly if the micro-organisms involved are especially virulent. Osteonecrosis occurs, together with suppuration, within the cancellous spaces of the bone.

More commonly, infections of dental origin do not remain localised within bone but pass from the confines of the bone into the soft tissues. This involves spread along lines of least resistance to the inflammatory process. Passage of an infection through the *cortical bony plate* tends to occur through thin cortical plates before thick cortex.

Having pierced the cortical plate, the further spread of infection is determined largely by tissue and fascial spaces which offer minimum resistance. The presence and arrangement of such spaces must be realised to understand how dental infections can spread throughout adjoining soft tissues and into more distant regions.

The *direction of spread* of dental infections into the soft tissues from the mandible and maxilla is dependent on the tooth or teeth involved and the site of perforation of the cortical plate relative to buccinator or mylohyoid muscle.

Infections entering soft tissues may remain localised, forming an abscess, or become diffuse — a cellulitis. Both are characterised by swelling. The circumscribed swelling related to an abscess is *fluctuant* if pus is present. Abscesses tend to 'point' and discharge upon a free surface such as the skin

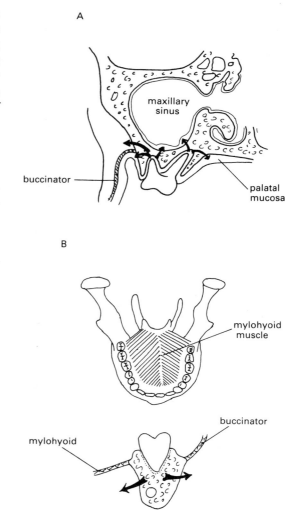

Fig. 1.6 A — Diagram showing the possible routes of spread of infection from an upper molar tooth. B — Possible routes of spread of infection from mandibular molar and premolar teeth.

or mucous membrane. The presence of pus is usually indicated by a yellowish head in the swelling. In contrast the diffuse swelling due to cellulitis is firm and brawny since no pus is present.

Spread of infections from various sites (Fig. 1.6)

1. *Maxillary anteriors*: infections tend to pass through the thin buccal cortical plate of the maxilla to enter the soft tissues of the face (see Ch. 5). Palatal spread can occur particularly if the tooth apex lies more palatally. Infections arising from lateral incisors after piercing the palatal bone track backwards beneath the firmly attached palatal mucosa to point at the junction of the hard and soft palates.

2. *Maxillary premolars*: infections pierce the thin buccal plate and either spread into the buccal sulcus or into the soft tissues of the face.

3. *Maxillary molar teeth*: infections may spread buccally into the soft tissues above or below buccinator muscle, or they may spread into the maxillary sinus or palatally to the palatal mucosa.

4. *Mandibular anteriors*: the apices of these teeth lie above the attachment of mylohyoid muscle. Lingual or labial spread may occur. *Lingual* spread results in infection of the sublingual tissue compartment above mylohyoid muscle. *Labial* spread can occur into the tissues lining the labial sulcus or downwards into the tissues of the chin.

5. *Mandibular premolars*: the apices of the premolars lie above mylohyoid attachment. Lingual spread of infection occurs into the sublingual compartment. Buccal spread is into the tissues of the buccal vestibule and soft tissues of the face.

6. *Mandibular molars*: the root apices of the second and third molars lie beneath the attachment of mylohyoid muscle. The first molar root apices usually lie above but this varies from individual to individual. Thus, infections from molar teeth may spread lingually into either the *sublingual* or *submandibular* tissue compartments. Buccal spread usually occurs below the level of attachment of buccinator muscle (the external oblique line) into the soft tissues of the face to lie outside the buccopharyngeal fascia. Spread of infection from the first molar tooth whose root apices may lie above the external oblique line does occur into the tissues of the buccal sulcus.

Further spread of infection is governed by adjoining fascial and tissue spaces (Ch. 7). However, while they may influence strongly the direction of spread of infection, it is prudent to remember that unexpected variations can occur.

2

Osteology 1: skull and skull bones

The osteology of the skull, and indeed of any region of the body, cannot be learnt merely by reading the text and looking at the diagrams in books. It is essential to have a skull in front of you and to identify the bones and named parts of bones as one reads through the textbook.

GENERAL CONSIDERATIONS

The skull is situated at the superior end of the vertebral column. It consists of two main parts. The *cranial part* lies posterosuperiorly and is a rigid bony box containing and protecting the brain and its coverings and other intracranial structures, including the middle and inner ears. Extending anteroinferiorly from the cranial part is the *facial skeleton* containing the cavities of the eyes, nose and mouth and supporting the teeth.

Cranial part. This is composed of frontal, parietal, temporal, occipital and sphenoid bones. Parts of these bones, except the parietal bones, form the *base* of the skull as well as the skull *vault*.

Facial skeleton. This is further divided into two parts — the *upper* and *lower* facial skeletons. The upper facial skeleton is related to the orbits, nose, palate and upper teeth. The bulk of it is formed by the maxilla which forms part of the orbital margin, much of the nasal cavity, and holds the upper (maxillary) teeth. Laterally it is attached to the zygomatic bone which forms a 'flying buttress' with the temporal bone. The lower facial skeleton is formed by the mandible, holding the lower (mandibular) teeth. It articulates with the temporal bone.

The bones of the skull are united by immobile fibrous joints known as *sutures*. The mandible, however, is mobile, and articulates at the synovial *temporomandibular joint* (TMJ).

Facial buttress system (Fig. 2.1)

During mastication considerable forces are generated between the upper and lower teeth. These are *vertical* loading forces and are transmitted through the facial skeleton and dissipated over the skull vault. The facial skeleton is mainly composed of light, hollow bones and certain regions are strengthened to withstand and transmit these forces forming the *facial buttress* system.

In the upper facial skeleton the *frontomaxillary*, *zygomatic* and *pterygopalatine* buttresses transmit force onto the skull vault. The lower border and oblique lines of the body and the posterior border of the ramus of the mandible are likewise strong and transmit force to the vault through the glenoid fossa of the temporal bone.

Age changes in the skull (Fig. 2.2)

During development the framework or outline of the skull bones is laid down either in cartilage or in membrane. The skull base is formed by the *chondrocranium* — a plate of cartilage which houses the developing ear and nasal systems. The vault develops in membrane as does the upper facial skeleton in relation to the outer wall of the nasal capsule. The mandible develops in membrane related to Meckel's cartilage.

Centres of ossification arise in certain areas within this framework and extend to produce the skull bones. Bones may arise from one or many

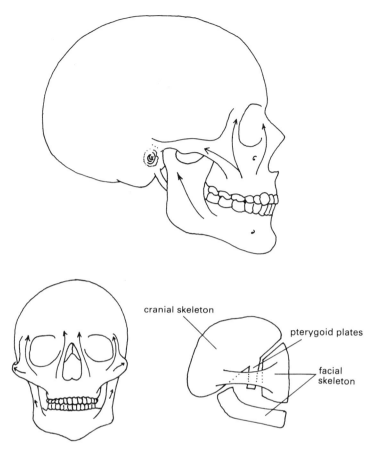

Fig. 2.1 The facial buttress system. The components of the cranial and facial skeletons are also shown diagrammatically (below right).

such centres. Fusion occurs at the junctions between ossification centres at various times, once growth at the junction is complete. Growth of the skull continues throughout fetal life into childhood and, in certain sites, into adulthood. Changes in the skull also occur in relation to advancing age.

Fetal skull

During the fetal period active growth occurs in most skull areas. Growth of the vault is rapid in the late fetal and early newborn period and is related to brain growth. The vault of the fetal skull is, therefore, relatively large in comparison with the facial skeleton. The bones of the vault are separated by linear sutures and, in places, by larger spaces known as *fontanelles*. The diamond-shaped

anterior fontanelle lies between the frontal bone (still in two halves separated by the *metopic* suture) anteriorly and the parietal bones posteriorly. The triangular *posterior* fontanelle lies between the parietal bones anteriorly and the occipital bone behind.

The orbits are also large, their vertical diameter being roughly equal to the height of the maxilla and mandible together. The maxilla is small, is packed with developing teeth, and lacks alveolar processes. The maxillary sinus is poorly developed. The mandible, also small, is in two halves separated at the mental symphysis. Its body also contains developing teeth and lacks alveolar processes. The mental foramen lies near its lower border and the angle formed by the body and the ramus is obtuse.

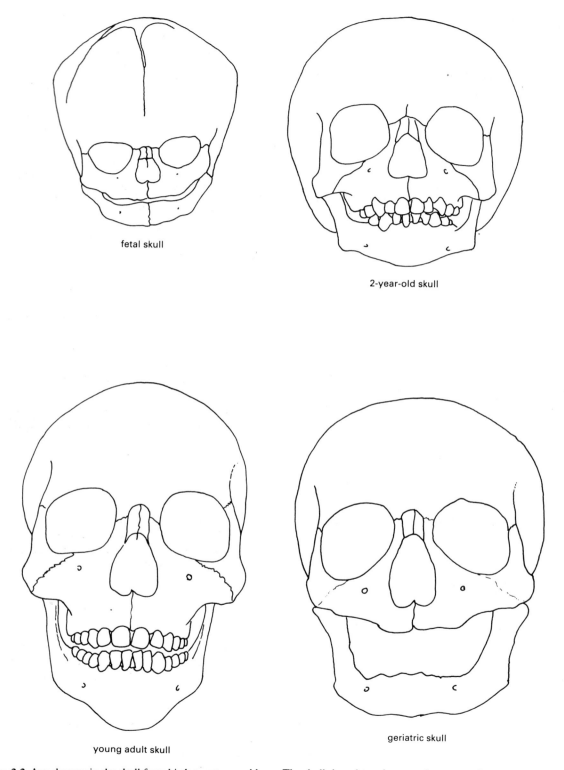

fetal skull

2-year-old skull

young adult skull

geriatric skull

Fig. 2.2 Age changes in the skull from birth to extreme old age. The skulls have been drawn to the same scale.

Adult skull

The posterior fontanelle has closed by the end of the first year of life and the anterior fontanelle by the end of the second year. The metopic suture fuses during the second year and by the tenth year the cranial vault has reached nearly adult size. The spheno-occipital synchondrosis of the cranial base continues to grow until about the sixteenth year and fuses by the twenty-fifth year. Continued growth of the facial skeleton leads to an increase in maxillary and mandibular height. Growth of the alveolar processes is related to the appearance and establishment of the dentition. The nasal cavity increases in height and the paranasal sinuses grow so that by adulthood the height of the maxilla and mandible is twice that of the orbit. The angle of the mandible is now nearly at a right angle, the symphysis has fused at the end of the first year, and the mental foramen lies halfway between upper and lower borders. Due to the development of the muscles the bones have become heavier and rougher and the facial buttresses are more prominent. With increasing age the sutures of the skull begin to fuse and disappear and the dentition may be lost with subsequent absorption of the alveolar processes of the maxilla and mandible. The mental foramen in the edentulous mandible lies nearer its upper border.

Sex differences

Adult female skulls are lighter, thinner and smaller than their male counterparts. However, in relation to the weight of the rest of the skeleton, the female skull is relatively larger.

The male skull appears rougher and more heavily ridged than the female and the zygomatic arches, mastoid processes and the external occipital protuberance are more prominent. The superciliary ridges are more prominent and rounded but the parietal eminences appear less marked than in the female. The male palate is wider.

Frontal bone (Fig. 2.3)

The frontal bone forms the forehead and anterior part of the cranium and is joined to the two parietal bones posteriorly by the *coronal* suture.

The bone is smoothly convex anteriorly and superiorly but is irregular inferiorly where it forms the superior margins of the orbits. In this area the bone is thickened and forms the *supraorbital ridges*, readily palpable in the living.

The irregularity of the lower border is caused by downward processes of bone which form part of the medial and lateral margins of the orbits. The medial process articulates with the frontal process of the maxilla and the lateral process with the frontal process of the zygomatic bone at the zygomaticofrontal suture. Between the frontal processes of the maxillae lie the nasal bones which articulate superiorly with the frontal bone at the *nasion*.

At the junction of the medial third and lateral two-thirds of the superior rim of the orbit lies the *supraorbital notch* or *foramen* through which passes the supraorbital nerve and vessels.

Extending horizontally backwards from the lower border are the twin *orbital plates* of the bone which form most of the roof of each orbit. They are separated by a gap in the midline which is completed by the ethmoid bone.

The frontal bone articulates inferolaterally with the greater wing of the sphenoid.

Within the anterior part of the bone above the nasion, lie the paired *frontal sinuses*. There is considerable individual variation in their size and shape.

Development

The frontal bone develops in membrane in two halves which fuse at about the fifth year but occasionally may fail to fuse totally leaving a persistent median suture in the adult called the *metopic* suture.

Parietal bone (Fig. 2.3)

These paired bones form much of the top, sides and back of the skull vault. The two parietal bones are quadrilateral in shape with convex outer surfaces. The areas of maximum convexity are known as the parietal *eminences*.

The bones articulate with one another in the midline at the *sagittal* suture, with the frontal bone anteriorly at the *coronal* suture, with the sphenoid bone inferolaterally forming part of the *pterion*,

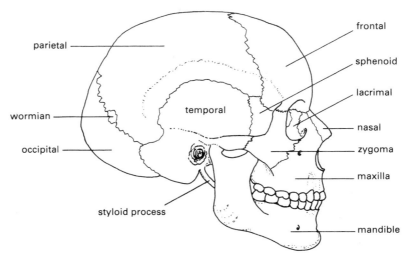

Fig. 2.3 Lateral view of skull.

with the temporal bone inferolaterally and with the occipital bone posteriorly at the *lambdoid suture*.

The outer surface of the bone is crossed in its lower third by the curved temporal ridges, the lower giving attachment to the temporalis muscle and the upper to the temporal fascia overlying the muscle. The inner surface shows grooves for the middle meningeal vessels and their branches running upward on the bone from its inferior edge. A groove running along the superior edge, more marked on the right, is for the *superior sagittal venous sinus*, with a series of depressions lateral to it for the *arachnoid granulations*. Occasionally there is a deep wide groove at the posteroinferior corner which marks the termination of the *transverse venous sinus*.

Development

The parietal bone develops in membrane from two centres located in the region of the parietal eminence.

In the fetal skull, with incomplete ossification, there are bony deficiences at the frontoparietal and occipitoparietal articulations. Anteriorly, where the sagittal, coronal and metopic sutures come together at the *bregma*, this deficiency is diamond-shaped and known as the *anterior fontanelle*. This closes fully at about 18 months of age. Posteriorly, where the sagittal and lambdoid sutures come to-

gether at the *lambda*, the bony deficiency is triangular and known as the *posterior fontanelle*. This closes 2–3 months after birth.

The widest part of the fetal skull — the biparietal diameter — lies between the parietal eminences.

Occipital bone (Fig. 2.4)

The occipital is a single bone which forms most of the posterior part of the cranial vault and the posterior part of the base of the skull.

The bone is trapezoidal in shape and both its outer and inner surfaces are markedly curved. The inferior part of the bone is pierced by the large *foramen magnum* which transmits the spinal cord and its coverings, the vertebral arteries and the XIth (spinal accessory) cranial nerves.

The occipital bone can be divided into four parts that lie around the foramen magnum. Anterior to the foramen is the *basilar* part or basiocciput. Posterior to the foramen lies the *squamous* part. On each side of the foramen lie the lateral or *condylar* parts.

The basilar part is thick and short and articulates anteriorly with the body of the sphenoid bone forming the *spheno-occipital synchondrosis*. On its undersurface, in the midline near the foramen, is the *pharyngeal tubercle* for the attachment of the posterior wall of the pharynx. The intracranial as-

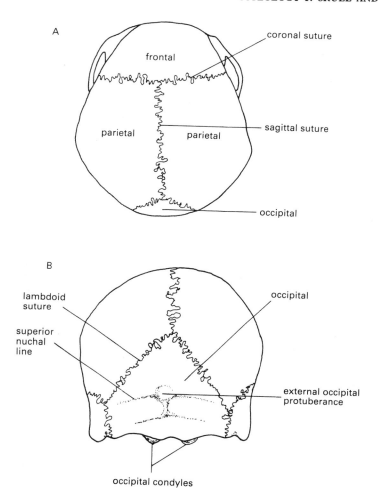

Fig. 2.4 A — Superior view of skull. B — Posterior view of skull.

pect is grooved and supports the medulla oblongata and vertebral arteries centrally and the lateral border has a half-groove, completed laterally by the petrous part of the temporal bone, for the inferior petrosal venous sinus.

The two lateral parts of the bone have, on their inferior surfaces, the occipital *condyles* which articulate with the atlas and permit the movements of nodding and some lateral rocking but not rotation. Opening anterolateral to each condyle is the *hypoglossal canal* which transmits the XIIth (hypoglossal) cranial nerve. Opening posterior to each condyle is the *posterior condylar foramen* which transmits an emissary vein.

Projecting laterally to each condyle are the *jugular processes* forming the posterior walls of the

jugular foramina through which pass the internal jugular veins, the inferior petrosal sinuses and the IXth, Xth and XIth (glossopharyngeal, vagus and accessory) cranial nerves. The anterior part of the jugular foramen is formed by the temporal bone.

At the outer end of the intracranial surface of each lateral part is a prominent process with a deep groove running sharply round it medially. Within it lies the sigmoid venous sinus.

The squamous part of the bone lies posterior to the foramen magnum and curves sharply upward to form the back of the cranial vault. It articulates with the squamous part of the temporal bones laterally and the parietal bones above.

On the lower part of its outer surface are the transverse *superior* and *inferior nuchal lines* and, in the midline, the palpable *external occipital pro-tuberance*. On the intracranial surface, at about its centre, is the *internal occipital protuberance*. Running downwards from it to the foramen magnum is the internal occipital *crest*, running laterally from it on both sides are grooves for the transverse sinuses and running upward, slightly to the right of midline, a groove for the superior sagittal sinus.

Development

The basilar, lateral and the lower part of the squamous parts (below the superior nuchal line) are laid down in cartilage and the rest of the bone in membrane. At birth the bone is in four portions; the squamous and lateral parts unite in the third year and these join the basilar part in the fourth to fifth years.

Temporal bone (Fig. 2.5)

These two bones form the lateral part of the cranial vault and part of the base of the skull. Each is composed of *squamous*, *petrous*, *tympanic* and *styloid* parts.

The squamous part is a thin plate of bone articulating superiorly with the parietal bone, anteriorly with the greater wing of the sphenoid and posteriorly with the occipital bone. It forms the upper part of the temporal bone. Projecting anteriorly from the lower part of the outer surface of the squamous part is a long arched bony process, the *zygomatic process*, which articulates anteriorly with the zygomatic bone. Below the root of the zygomatic process is the *mandibular fossa* which receives the mandibular condyle, forming the *temporomandibular* joint. The mandibular fossa is continuous anteriorly with an eminence, the *articular tubercle*, projecting downwards from the root of the zygomatic process.

The mandibular fossa is in two parts, the anterior formed by the squamous part of the temporal bone and the posterior portion by the tympanic part of the temporal bone. The two parts are divided by the *squamotympanic fissure* which transmits the tympanic branch of the maxillary artery and the chorda tympani branch of the VIIth (facial) cranial nerve. Posterior to the fossa lies the *external auditory meatus*.

The outer surface of the squamous part is smoothly convex but a curved ridge may be visible posteriorly for attachment of the dense temporal fascia. The inner surface is concave and has well-marked grooves for the branches of the middle meningeal artery. It joins the petrous part of the bone inferiorly at the *petrosquamous* suture.

The tympanic part of the temporal bone forms the posterior, nonarticulating, part of the mandibular fossa and the anterior wall and floor of the bony external auditory meatus. Its inferior part is closely adjacent to the front of the styloid process and has a sharp inferior edge, the *vaginal process*.

The petrous part of the temporal bone, named thus because of its hardness, is wedge-shaped and lies at the base of the skull between the sphenoid and occipital bones. It contains within it the middle and inner ears.

The *mastoid process*, the outer, inferior and posterior portion of the petrous part, projects downwards behind the bony external auditory meatus. It is rough and gives rise to the sternomastoid muscle. On its inner aspect is a deep groove for the attachment of digastric muscle and medial and parallel to this is the *occipital groove* for the occipital artery as it runs backward towards the occiput. At the anterior end of the digastric groove, just behind the styloid process, is the *stylomastoid foramen* which transmits the VIIth (facial) cranial nerve. Lying posterior to the mastoid process is the *mastoid foramen* which transmits a vein to the sigmoid venous sinus which grooves the intracranial aspect of the process.

The mastoid process contains many cellular spaces, the *mastoid air cells*, which open into the middle ear through the mastoid antrum and aditus. The antrum is closely related to the posterior cranial fossa, the temporal lobe of the brain and the sigmoid venous sinus and separated from them by a thin bony plate. The air cells, and hence the mastoid process itself, are not present at birth but enlarge during puberty to attain prominence in the adult.

The apex of the wedge of the petrous temporal bone is directed inwards and forwards and articulates between the greater wing of the sphenoid anteriorly and the basilar part of the occipital bone posteriorly. The base of the wedge is applied to the squamous part of the bone at the petrosquamous

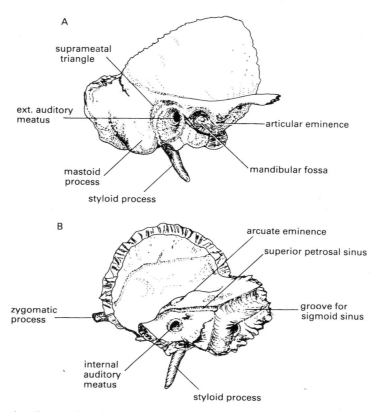

Fig. 2.5 Temporal bone. A — Lateral view of right temporal bone. B — Medial view of right temporal bone.

suture. The petrous part has anterior, posterior and inferior surfaces.

On the anterior surface, at the apex, is a depression in which lies the trigeminal ganglion of the Vth (trigeminal) cranial nerve. Below this is the internal opening of the *carotid canal*. Lateral to the apex is the rounded *arcuate eminence* which indicates the position of the superior semicircular canal within the bone. Anterior to the eminence are two foramina, one anterolateral to the other, from which parallel grooves run towards the apex.

Passing through the larger, posteromedial, foramen is the greater petrosal nerve which runs in its groove to the *foramen lacerum*, whose posterior boundary is formed by the anterior part of the apex of the bone. Through the smaller foramen passes the lesser petrosal nerve which runs within its groove towards the foramen ovale of the sphenoid bone.

Between the arcuate eminence and the foramina

is the area of bone which forms the roof of the tympanic cavity, the *tegmen tympani*.

The posterior surface of the petrous part forms part of the posterior cranial fossa. At about its centre is a large foramen, the *internal auditory meatus*, which is directed laterally and through which passes the VIIth (facial) cranial nerve, the VIIIth (auditory) cranial nerve and the auditory branch of the basilar artery (the labyrinthine artery). Lateral to the meatus is a narrow slit, the *vestibular aqueduct*, containing the terminal part of the endolymphatic duct.

On the border between the anterior and posterior surfaces is a groove for the superior petrosal venous sinus. A half-groove, completed by the occipital bone, runs along the inferior border of the posterior surface near the apex. In this lies the inferior petrosal venous sinus.

The inferior surface of the petrous part forms part of the base of the skull. Near the apex the bone is roughened and gives partial origin to levator palati and tensor tympani muscles. Lateral to this is a depression in which lies the auditory tube, directed forwards and inwards. Behind and lateral to this area is the large circular opening of the *carotid canal* which transmits the internal carotid artery. The canal is vertical in its first part but bends at right angles to run horizontally forwards and inwards emerging, as seen, at the apex of the bone. Posterior to it is part of the deep *jugular fossa*, completed posteriorly by the occipital bone and lodging the bulb of the internal jugular vein. The foramen also transmits the inferior petrosal venous sinus and the IXth (glossopharyngeal), Xth (vagus) and XIth (spinal accessory) cranial nerves. On the bony crest dividing the jugular fossa and the external opening of the carotid canal is a small foramen which transmits the tympanic branch of the glossopharyngeal nerve.

Lying lateral to the jugular fossa is the *styloid process*. This bony process projects downwards, forwards and inwards; is usually about two centimetres long but varies in size, shape and length from person to person.

Development

The temporal bone develops from its four main parts. The squamous and tympanic parts ossify in membrane from a single centre each, the squamous at about the second month, the tympanic at about the third month. The petrous part ossifies in cartilage from four or more centres in the fifth month and the styloid process ossifies in

cartilage from two centres; one for the base of the process appears shortly before birth and the other shortly after birth.

The squamous and tympanic parts join shortly before birth. The basal centre of the styloid joins the petrous part during the first year of life. The petrous part joins the squamous and tympanic parts at about the same time. The distal styloid centre joins the basal centre after puberty but in some cases, never.

Sphenoid bone (Fig. 2.6)

This bone is single, situated at the base of the skull, and consists of a central *body* from which two pairs of wings, the *greater* and *lesser wings*, project laterally and from which two paired plates of bone, the *pterygoid processes*, project downward.

The body of the sphenoid is roughly cuboidal in shape with anterior, posterior, superior and inferior surfaces.

The anterior surface presents a midline ridge, the *ethmoidal crest*, which articulates with the perpendicular plate of the ethmoid bone. In the adult the body of the sphenoid is almost completely hollowed out by the paired sphenoidal *air sinuses* whose openings lie on either side of the ethmoidal crest closed in by the thin plates of the sphenoidal *turbinal* bones through which they communicate with the nasal cavity.

The posterior surface of the body articulates with the occipital bone at the *spheno-occipital synchondrosis*.

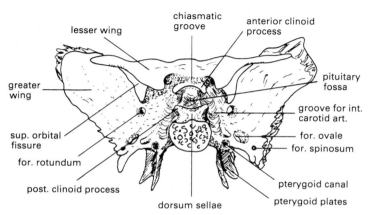

Fig. 2.6 Superior view of sphenoid bone.

The superior surface has, anteriorly, the *ethmoidal spine* which articulates with the cribriform plate of the ethmoid bone. Behind this is a smooth flat area, the *sphenoidal jugum*, and behind this the transverse *chiasmatic groove* stretching laterally on either side to the *optic canals* which transmit the IInd (optic) cranial nerves and the ophthalmic arteries. Posterior to the groove is a small tubercle and behind this a deep hollow housing the pituitary gland, the *pituitary fossa*.

Anterolateral to the fossa on each side are the *anterior clinoid processes*, thick posterior projections of bone from the bases of the lesser wings. Their medial edges are smoothly curved to form bony semicircles in which sit the internal carotid arteries. A broad groove for these arteries can be traced downwards from the anterior clinoid processes, horizontally backwards past the pituitary fossa on either side, and then again downwards to the point at which they enter the cranial cavity. At the most posterior part of the groove, between it and the greater wing, is a small projection of bone, the *lingula*.

The vertical posterior wall of the pituitary fossa is formed by a square plate of bone, the *dorsum sellae*, from whose upper angles project the two *posterior clinoid processes* which tend to overhang and deepen the fossa. The posterior surface of the dorsum sellae slopes downwards and backwards to the spheno-occipital synchondrosis and supports the pons. The dorsum sellae is notched on either side by the VIth (abducens) cranial nerves. The area that is formed by the pituitary fossa, the dorsum sellae and the anterior and posterior clinoid processes is known as the *sella turcica* because of its fancied resemblance to a Turkish saddle.

The inferior surface of the body is flat with a thick midline ridge of bone which articulates below with a groove between the alae of the vomer and ends anteriorly in the prominent *rostrum*. The alae are, in turn, held in place by the *vaginal processes* which turn inward from the bases of the medial pterygoid plates, and partly overlap the inferior surface.

The lesser wings of the sphenoid are composed of two triangular plates of bone which project horizontally outwards from the upper anterior part of the body. The base of this triangle is attached to the body by two roots. The upper root is flat, horizontal, and merges into the jugum; the lower root is thicker and set obliquely into the side of the body lower down. The two roots enclose the optic canals. The apex of the triangle is sharp, the upper surface is smooth and flat and the lower surface forms the posterior part of the roof of the orbit and the upper border of the *superior orbital fissure*.

The fissure is triangular in shape, bounded above by the lesser wing and below by part of the greater wing of the sphenoid and transmits, from lateral to medial, the lacrimal, frontal, trochlear and abducens nerves, the superior division of the oculomotor nerve, the nasociliary nerve, the inferior division of the oculomotor nerve, the orbital branch of the middle meningeal artery and the ophthalmic veins.

The lesser wing articulates with the frontal bone anteriorly. The posterior border of the wing is free and continues medially into the anterior clinoid process. Along this border runs the sphenoparietal venous sinus, joining the cavernous sinus under cover of the anterior clinoid process.

The greater wings of the sphenoid curve outward and upward from the body. They are deeply concave on their intracranial surfaces and form part of the middle cranial fossa. The outer ends of the wings form part of the lateral skull vault.

Three pairs of foramina are visible on the intracranial surface. Anteriorly, just below the medial end of the superior orbital fissure, lies the circular *foramen rotundum*. It is directed forwards and slightly outwards and transmits the maxillary division of the Vth (trigeminal) cranial nerve. Posterolateral to this is the large oval *foramen ovale* which transmits the mandibular division of the Vth cranial nerve, the accessory meningeal artery and occasionally the lesser superficial petrosal nerve. (This nerve occasionally passes through a separate foramen which lies medial to the foramen spinosum.) The third foramen lies posterolateral to the foramen ovale in the most posterior part of the greater wing and is the small, circular, *foramen spinosum* transmitting the middle meningeal artery and the middle meningeal branch of the mandibular nerve.

The upper border of the greater wing forms the inferior margin of the superior orbital fissure medially and lateral to this articulates with the frontal bone. The extreme outer edge of the wing is bevelled and articulates with the parietal bone at the *pterion*. From this area the lateral border of the wing curves downwards and then backwards and articulates with the squamous temporal bone.

The lateral border ends in a well-marked downward projection, the *spinous process*, to which are attached the tensor palati muscle and the internal lateral ligament of the mandible.

Lying between the spinous process and the body of the sphenoid is the posterior border whose outer half articulates with the petrous temporal bone and whose inner half forms the anterior boundary of the foramen lacerum.

The outer surface of the greater wing possesses three distinct areas, the *orbital, temporal and infratemporal* surfaces.

The orbital surface is quadrilateral, almost flat, faces anteromedially, and forms part of the posterior and lateral walls of the orbit. It is bounded medially by the superior orbital fissure, above by an area which articulates with the frontal bone and laterally by a ridge articulating with the zygomatic bone. Below is a rounded border forming the upper edge of the *inferior orbital fissure* (the maxilla forms the lower edge) which transmits the maxillary division of the Vth cranial nerve and its zygomatic branch. The fissure communicates medially with the *pterygopalatine fossa* and laterally with the *infratemporal fossa*.

The temporal surface is also quadrilateral and faces laterally. It articulates anteriorly with the zygomatic bone, above with the frontal and parietal bones and posteriorly with the squamous temporal bone. The surface is concave anteroposteriorly and gives attachment to temporalis muscle. Its inferior border is bounded by a bony ridge, the *infratemporal crest*, which separates it from the infratemporal surface.

The infratemporal surface faces downward and forms the roof of the infratemporal fossa.

The *pterygoid processes* project downward from the junction of the body and the greater wings of the sphenoid. Each process is formed of two plates of bone, the *medial* and *lateral pterygoid plates*, which are joined anteriorly, except in their lower part where they are separated by the *pterygoid notch*. The plates diverge from each other

posteriorly creating a deep space, the *pterygoid fossa*, between them. This is separated above, by an oblique ridge, from the smaller, shallower, *scaphoid fossa*, giving origin to tensor palati muscle. The tuberosity of the palatine bone fills in the pterygoid notch in the articulated skull.

The lateral pterygoid plate is thin and flat with a sharp projection on its posterior edge, the pterygospinous process. Its medial and lateral surfaces give origin to the medial and lateral pterygoid muscles, respectively.

The medial pterygoid plate is thicker, articulates anteriorly with the palatine bone to form the lateral wall of the posterior part of the nasal cavity, and curves inferiorly into a hook of bone, the *pterygoid hamulus*. The lower half of its posterior border gives rise to superior constrictor muscle with the pharyngeal end of the pharyngotympanic tube above it. Attached to the hamulus is the *pterygomandibular raphé* and winding around its lateral part is the tendon of tensor palati muscle.

Above and medial to the scaphoid fossa lies the *pterygoid* or *Vidian canal*. It arises at the anterior part of the foramen lacerum and passes forwards through the fused bases of the pterygoid plates to open into the pterygopalatine fossa. It transmits the nerve of the canal, formed by the union of the greater superficial petrosal and deep petrosal nerves, and a branch of the maxillary artery.

Development

The body, the lesser wings and the medial parts of the greater wings develop in cartilage; the rest of the bone, except for the hamuli, develops in membrane.

The bone is divided into two parts. The *presphenoid*, which consists of the anterior part of the body and the lesser wings and the *postsphenoid* consisting of the posterior part of the body, the greater wings, and the pterygoid processes.

Centres of ossification appear at about the eighth intrauterine week. The pre- and postsphenoid parts of the body unite at about the eighth month and at birth the sphenoid is in three parts; the body with the lesser wings forming one part and the greater wings and pterygoid processes on either side, the other two parts. These fuse at about one year after birth. The turbinate bones join the body between the tenth and twelfth years and are completely fused at about the twentieth year. Finally, the sphenoid joins the occipital bone between the eighteenth to the twenty-fifth years.

Nasal bone

The two nasal bones form the bony upper part of the nose and lie below the frontal bone, one on each side of the midline. Their size and shape vary from person to person but they are small and possess four borders and two surfaces.

The upper border is thick and narrow and articulates above with the frontal bone at the *nasion*. The medial borders of the bones are straight, meet in the midline, and have a slight crest on their inner surfaces which forms part of the nasal septum and articulates from above downwards with the nasal spine of the frontal bone, the perpendicular plate of the ethmoid and the nasal septal cartilage.

The lateral border articulates with the frontal process of the maxilla and the thin lower border inclines obliquely downwards, outwards and backwards to provide attachment for the alar cartilage of the nose.

Both outer and inner surfaces are fairly smooth, the inner bearing a vertical groove in which lies a branch of the anterior ethmoidal nerve.

Development

Each bone develops in membrane from one centre which appears at about the eighth week of fetal life.

Vomer

The vomer is a single bone forming part of the nasal septum.

The bone is wedge-shaped with superior, inferior, posterior and anterosuperior borders. The bulk of the bone is made of two fused plates and is flat.

The superior border is thickened and here the plates splay outwards to form the *alae* which receive part of the body of the sphenoid between them. The alae are overlapped by the vaginal pro-

cesses of the medial pterygoid plates of the sphenoid.

The posterior border is thin and curved and forms the posterior edge of the nasal septum. The inferior border articulates with the midline crest on the upper surface of the palatal bones posteriorly, and the maxilla anteriorly.

The anterosuperior border consists of two laminae of bone separated by a groove. In the upper half of this groove these laminae receive between them the perpendicular plate of the ethmoid bone; and in the lower half the septal cartilage of the nose.

The lateral surfaces of the bone are smooth, with well-defined grooves seen on both sides running roughly parallel to the anterosuperior border. In these run the nasopalatine vessels. The best-defined groove, sometimes a canal, lodges the nasopalatine nerve.

Development

At about the ninth week of fetal life a centre of ossification appears on either side of the postero-inferior edge of the septal plate of the cartilaginous nasal capsule. These centres extend to form the two laminae of bone, the cartilage enclosed between them being the *vomerine cartilage*, and join with each other to form a Y-shaped trough of bone along the lower edge of the septal cartilage.

The bone increases in size and, at about the fourth month, begins to articulate with the body of the sphenoid. At about seven years of age ossification in the perpendicular plate of the ethmoid extends to the vomer and the two bones unite behind the cartilaginous septum, but coalescence of the two laminae is not complete until after puberty. After middle age the ethmoid and vomer are usually fused together.

Zygomatic bone

These two small bones form the prominence of the cheek, part of the floor and lateral wall of the orbit, and contribute to the temporal fossa and the zygomatic arch.

Each bone has a body with four processes. The *frontal*, *maxillary* and *temporal* processes all lie in roughly the same curved plane and the *orbital* process projects almost at right angles inwards from it.

The external surface of the bone is smooth and convex. Near its centre are one or two foramina for the facial branches of the zygomatic nerve. Radiating upwards is the frontal process, whose rounded anterior border forms the lower lateral margin of the orbit, articulating superiorly with the frontal bone. Passing forwards and slightly inwards to form part of the floor and infraorbital margin is the maxillary process which articulates with the zygomatic process of the maxilla. Passing backwards to articulate with the zygomatic process of the temporal bone and complete the zygomatic arch is the temporal process. The inferior border of the temporal process is rough and gives origin to masseter muscle.

The orbital process projects inwards and backwards from the orbital margin. It forms part of the lateral wall of the orbit and separates it from the temporal fossa. It articulates with the greater wing of the sphenoid bone.

The internal surface, anteriorly, forms part of the lateral wall and floor of the orbit and shows one or two foramina for the passage of the zygomaticofacial nerves. Below the orbital plate is a rough area which articulates with the maxilla, and posteriorly the bone is relatively smooth and forms part of the temporal fossa. In this area are foramina for the zygomaticotemporal nerves.

Development

The bone develops in membrane from one centre appearing in the eighth week of life. Other centres may be present and occasionally the bone is seen to be in two parts, an upper and a lower.

Inferior turbinate bone

These paired bones form part of the lateral walls of the nasal cavity.

Each is a thin, curved plate of bone projecting medially downwards into the nose and forms the floor of the middle meatus and the roof of the inferior meatus.

Each bone has upper and lower borders, a sharp posterior end, and a more rounded anterior end.

The upper border is thin, irregular, and pos-

sesses three processes in its middle part by which it is attached to the nasal wall. Anteriorly the bone articulates with the maxilla and posteriorly with the palatal bone. Of the three processes, the anterior is a small, pointed *lacrimal process* projecting upward to articulate with the anteroinferior part of the lacrimal bone and forming the medial wall of the nasolacrimal canal below it. Centrally the large *maxillary process* is directed downwards from the superior edge of the bone and fits into the lower part of the opening of the maxillary antrum, articulating inferiorly with its edges. An upward extension from the posterior part of the maxillary process forms the posterior *ethmoidal process* which articulates superiorly with the uncinate process of the ethmoid bone.

The free lower border is thick, rough and pierced by numerous foraminae through which pass the vessels of the mucous membrane which covers the bone during life.

Development

A single centre for each bone appears in the fifth to sixth month of fetal life in the inturned lower edge of the lateral wall of the nasal capsule. This extends to form the inferior turbinate bone.

Lacrimal bone

These two small fragile bones lie at the anterior part of the medial wall of the orbit.

The bones are almost flat plates with *orbital* and *nasal* surfaces. The orbital surface articulates above with the frontal bone, behind with the ethmoid bone and in front with the frontal process of the maxilla. This surface is divided into a smaller anterior and a larger posterior part by a vertical ridge known as the *lacrimal crest*.

The anterior portion, together with the part of the frontal process of the maxilla lying anterior to it, forms a deep depression, the lacrimal *fossa*, visible just inside the medial margin of the orbit. The lacrimal fossa lodges the lacrimal sac above and the nasolacrimal duct in its lower part. A process of bone extends downwards from the fossa to form the medial wall of the duct articulating below with the inferior turbinate bone.

The posterior part of the orbital surface is smooth and forms part of the medial orbital wall.

The nasal surface is convex anteriorly, corresponding to the lacrimal fossa on the orbital surface, and smooth posteriorly. It forms part of the lateral wall of the nose and closes in the anterior ethmoidal air cells and partially helps close in the maxillary antrum. The inferior border articulates anteriorly with the inferior turbinate bone and posteriorly with the orbital plate of the maxilla.

Development

The lacrimal bone develops in membrane from one centre before the end of the third intrauterine month. It is closely related to the cartilage of the nasal capsule.

Ethmoid bone

The ethmoid bone lies between the orbital plates of the frontal bone with the body of the sphenoid bone behind and the maxilla below. It is a box-like bone and forms part of the anterior cranial fossa, part of the walls of the nasal cavity and part of the medial orbital wall.

The bone consists of three parts; a horizontal *cribriform plate*, a *perpendicular plate* and two *lateral cell masses*.

The cribriform plate is situated in the *ethmoid notch* between the orbital plates of the frontal bone. It is deeply grooved on either side to receive the olfactory bulbs and pierced by numerous small foramina which transmit olfactory nerve filaments from the olfactory mucous membrane of the nasal cavities. The body of the sphenoid bone articulates with the posterior part of the plate. Anteriorly, in the midline, is a triangular upward projection of bone, the *crista galli*, whose base articulates with the frontal bone anteriorly forming the posterior wall of the *foramen caecum* which may transmit a vein from the superior sagittal sinus to the nasal roof.

The perpendicular plate projects downwards in the midline from the undersurface of the cribriform plate and forms part of the nasal septum. Anteriorly this plate articulates with the frontal bones above and the nasal bones below, posteriorly with the sphenoid above and the vomer below, and inferiorly with the septal cartilage of the nose.

The two lateral cell masses consist of a number of thin-walled bony cavities, the *ethmoidal air cells*, which lie between two vertical bony plates. The inner plate forms part of the lateral wall of the nose. In its upper part a curved plate of bone protrudes into the nasal cavity as the *superior turbinate process*; below lies the rough free edge of the plate which curves outwards as the *middle turbinate process*. Between the two processes is a fissure, the *middle meatus*, and above the superior turbinate another, the *superior meatus*.

The outer bony plate, the *os planum*, forms part of the medial wall of the orbit and articulates with the frontal, lacrimal, maxillary, sphenoid and palatine bones. On its upper border are two bony canals, the *anterior* and *posterior ethmoidal canals*, which open into the orbit and transmit the ethmoidal nerves and arteries. Projecting downwards and backwards below the os planum is the *uncinate process* which partially closes in the orifice of the maxillary antrum and articulates with the inferior turbinate bone.

The ethmoidal air cells are divided into two sets which do not communicate with one another. The *anterior* ethmoidal cells communicate with the frontal sinus and open into the middle meatus through the *infundibulum*. The *posterior* ethmoidal cells open into the superior meatus and may communicate with the sphenoid air cells.

Development

The ethmoid develops from three centres, one for the perpendicular plate and one each for the lateral masses. The centres for the lateral masses are the first to appear, during the fifth intrauterine month, and at birth are ossified, although small and undeveloped. During the first year after birth a centre for the crista galli and the perpendicular plate appears and joins the lateral masses between the second and fifth years. The cribriform plate develops partly fron the perpendicular plate and partly from the lateral masses. The air cells begin to form at four to five years.

Palatine bone

The two palatine bones are situated towards the back of the nasal cavity, wedged between the maxilla and the pterygoid processes of the sphenoid bone. Each forms part of the lateral wall and floor of the nasal cavity, the roof of the mouth and the orbital floor.

Each bone is roughly L-shaped. The shorter limb forms the *horizontal* or *palatine plate*, the longer limb forms the *perpendicular* or *nasal plate*.

The horizontal plate is quadrilateral in shape. Its smooth upper surface forms the most posterior part of the floor of the nasal cavity. The rougher undersurface forms the back of the hard palate and gives rise to some of the palatal muscles and the palatal aponeurosis.

The anterior border is rough and articulates with the palatal process of the maxilla. The medial border is also rough, articulates in the midline with the horizontal plate of the opposite side, and has a raised crest on its nasal surface which supports the vomer. The posterior border is free, concave, gives origin to the soft palate, and has the *posterior nasal spine* projecting posteriorly in the midline. The lateral border curves smoothly into the perpendicular plate almost at right angles.

The thin perpendicular plate is irregularly shaped with *nasal* and *maxillary* surfaces, anterior and posterior borders. It ends above in two processes, the *orbital process* anteriorly and the *sphenoidal process* posteriorly. Protruding posterolaterally from the base of the plate is the *tuberosity* or *pyramidal process*.

The nasal surface is smooth but is divided into upper and lower parts by a horizontal ridge, the *conchal crest*, which articulates with the inferior turbinate bone. Below this the bone forms part of the inferior meatus; above, part of the middle meatus. Above this area may be another horizontal ridge, the *ethmoidal crest*, which articulates with the middle turbinate. The part of the plate above this forms part of the superior meatus.

The maxillary surface is rough and irregular and articulates with the maxilla. The bone is thin anteriorly and this border helps to close in the posterior part of the maxillary antrum and overlaps the part of the maxilla which lies anterior to it. Posteriorly the plate is thicker and shows the deep vertical *palatine groove* which forms the *palatine*

canal when it is articulated with the maxilla. The canal transmits the palatine vessels and nerves and opens onto the hard palate as the *greater palatine foramen*.

The posterior border of the plate is thick and grooved. The edges of the groove articulate with the pterygoid plates and the groove itself forms part of the pterygoid fossa. The pyramidal process fits into the pterygoid notch. On its undersurface are the *lesser palatine foramina* which vary in number and transmit the lesser palatine nerves and vessels.

Superiorly, the perpendicular plate ends in two processes. The anterior *orbital process* is directed upwards and outwards and articulates anterolaterally with the maxilla, anteromedially with the ethmoid and posteriorly with the sphenoid bone. Its upper surface forms part of the orbital floor, lying between the ethmoid and the maxilla.

The *sphenoidal process* is directed upwards and inwards and articulates with the sphenoid bone at the base of the medial pterygoid plate. The processes are separated by the deep *sphenopalatine notch*, converted into the *sphenopalatine foramen* by articulation above with the sphenoidal turbinate. It transmits nasal branches from the maxillary nerve and artery from the pterygopalatine fossa to the nasal cavity.

Development

The palatine bone develops in membrane from one centre on the inner side of the nasal capsule. Ossification begins in the second intrauterine month, extending inwards and upwards to form the horizontal and perpendicular plates respectively, and downwards to form the pyramidal process.

At first the bone is separated from the maxilla by the cartilage of the nasal capsule. As this atrophies the palatine bone comes to overlie the inner aspect of the maxilla and to fill in the maxillary antrum.

At birth the perpendicular and horizontal plates are about the same length, giving the nasal cavity a relatively small vertical measurement.

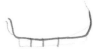

3

Osteology II: mandible and maxilla

MAXILLA (Fig. 3.1)

The maxillary bones form the upper jaw and much of the facial skeleton contributing to the orbital, nasal and oral cavities.

Each maxilla has a *body* and four processes, the *zygomatic*, *frontal*, *palatal* and *alveolar* processes. The body is shaped like a three-sided pyramid with the *nasal* surface forming the base, the *zygomatic process* the apex, and whose sides are the anterior *facial* surface, the *posterior* (infratemporal) surface and the superior *orbital* surface. It is hollow and contains the large *maxillary air sinus* or *antrum* which opens into the nasal cavity.

The orbital surface is smooth but is grooved posteriorly by the *infraorbital groove* passing forwards to the *infraorbital canal* which lies within the bone, opens onto the facial surface as the *infraorbital foramen* about 1 cm below the middle of the orbital margin and transmits the infraorbital nerve and vessels. It forms the roof of the maxillary air sinus and the orbital floor, articulates medially with the lacrimal and ethmoid bones and forms, posteriorly, the lower border of the *inferior orbital fissure*.

The facial surface is directed anterolaterally and is bounded by the alveolar process inferiorly, the orbital margin above, the external nasal aperture medially and laterally by the zygomatic process. The surface is ridged by the roots of the teeth and presents two concavities.

1. The *incisive fossa* above the incisor teeth with the *anterior nasal spine* medially and the eminence of the canine root laterally.

2. The larger *canine fossa* above the premolar teeth between the canine eminence and the zygomatic process.

The posterior surface is rounded and forms the anterior wall of the *infratemporal fossa* laterally and of the *pterygopalatine fossa* medially. It is separated from the lateral pterygoid plate by the *pterygomaxillary fissure* and is rough inferiorly where it articulates with the tuberosity of the palatine bone. Small *alveolar foramina* seen in this area transmit

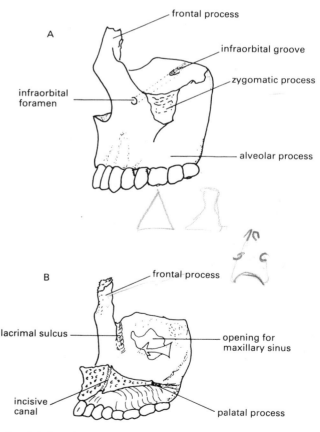

Fig. 3.1 A — Lateral aspect of left maxilla. B — Medial aspect of right maxilla.

the posterior superior alveolar (dental) nerves and vessels. Above, the posterior surface curves continuously into the orbital surface.

The nasal surface is flat, almost vertical, and shows, centrally, the large irregular opening into the maxillary sinus. This large opening visible in the disarticulated and dried bone is considerably reduced in size in the living by other bones and mucous membrane overlying it.

Posterior to the opening the surface is rough and overlain by the vertical plate of the palatine bone which closes in the posterior third of the opening. An oblique groove, the *greater palatine sulcus*, in this area, is converted into the *palatine canal* by the palatine bone. The upper part of the opening is closed in by the ethmoid bone, its lower part by the inferior turbinate and its upper anterior part by the lacrimal bone which closes in the deep *lacrimal sulcus* converting it into the *nasolacrimal canal* just anterior to the upper part of the opening.

The frontal process projects upwards from the body of the maxilla to articulate above with the frontal bone, anteriorly with the nasal bone and posteriorly with the lacrimal bone.

Its outer surface is smooth but bears a vertical ridge near its posterior border. This is the *anterior lacrimal crest* — a continuation medially of the lower orbital margin. The bone lying behind this forms part of the medial wall of the *lacrimal fossa* and *nasolacrimal canal*.

The inner surface of the process is also smooth, lies anterior to the lacrimal sulcus and is divided by a horizontal crest into upper and lower parts. The anterior end of the inferior turbinate bone articulates with this crest, the bone below it being related to the inferior meatus and the bone above to the middle and superior meatuses of the nose.

The zygomatic process articulates laterally with the zygomatic bone, separates the facial from the infratemporal areas of the bone and has an inferior ridge which extends down to the alveolar process between the first and second molars.

The palatal process projects inwards from the lower part of the body just above the alveolar process. It articulates with its fellow in the midline to form the bulk of the hard palate and has a midline crest to which the vomer is attached. Its posterior border articulates with the horizontal plate of the palatine bone. The upper surface is smooth

but the process is roughened below and shows a groove in the angle between it and the alveolar process in which the nerves and vessels emerging from the greater palatine foramen run.

On the upper surface anteriorly lie the twin *incisive canals* which transmit branches of the maxillary division of the trigeminal nerve, of the nasopalatine nerve and of the maxillary artery. The canals open onto the lower surface at the midline *incisive foramen*. A small suture may be seen running from the incisive foramen towards the lateral incisor and canine teeth; this separates the maxilla behind from the *premaxilla*.

The alveolar process hangs from the body of the maxilla and contains the sockets or *dental alveoli* for the upper teeth. It is gently curved and with the process of the opposite side forms a semi-ellipse, the maximum convexity lying anteriorly. Its outer surface is continuous with the outer surface of the body of the maxilla and its inner surface with the roof of the mouth. In its posterior part it forms the floor of the maxillary sinus and the roots of the upper teeth may project into the sinus. The rounded posterior part of the process may be called the *tuberosity* of the maxilla.

The sockets of the teeth cause prominences — *alveolar juga* — on the outer surface of the process. The alveoli for the incisors lie below the nasal opening, those for the canine, premolar and first molar teeth lie below the facial surface and those for the remaining two molars lie below the posterior surface posterior to the zygomatic process. The alveoli are separated from each other by thin walls of bone — the *interalveolar septa*. Within the alveoli lie the *interradicular septa* — bony walls which form separate chambers for each root of each tooth.

Development

The maxilla develops in membrane in two parts, one lying on the outer side of the nasal capsule in the maxillary process of the mandibular arch, the other — the premaxilla — in the frontonasal process. Early fusion of the two parts is characteristic of the human face.

Ossification starts at six weeks in utero in the region of the future canine and spreads back towards the zygomatic bone and forwards towards the premaxilla. From this strip of bone growth upwards forms the frontal process and growth downwards forms the lateral alveolar plate.

The palatal processes form and fuse by the ninth week, ossification extending into them by the tenth week. The area of bone anterior to the incisive foramen and suture is premaxillary and formed from the frontonasal process.

Downward growth from the outer parts of the palatal processes forms the medial alveolar plate. The bony trough formed by the medial and lateral alveolar plates is divided later into the alveoli by septa growing between them.

Secondary cartilage appears in the area of the zygomatic process at about eight weeks in utero and grows rapidly for a time.

At birth the maxilla differs from its adult appearance. Its vertical height is smaller in proportion (due to the smallness of the maxillary sinus) and the alveolar process is small. The maxillary sinus begins as an outward-growing pouch in the third month and at birth is a small depression on the medial side of the body of the maxilla. It grows steadily in size, its roof reaching the infraorbital canal in the first year and then grows fairly rapidly with the bone up to about the ninth year and more slowly from then on. Its form alters as the permanent teeth erupt, the floor of the sinus gradually falling to and then below the level of the floor of the nose.

MANDIBLE (Fig. 3.2)

The mandible forms the lower part of the skeleton of the face and carries the lower teeth. It is mobile, unlike the other skull bones described, and gives insertion and origin to some important muscle groups, notably the muscles of mastication and of the tongue.

The bone consists of two halves, fused at the midline *symphysis*. Each half has a *body* and a *ramus*; the *angle* of the jaw being the prominence where the lower, subcutaneous, border of the body joins the posterior border of the ramus.

Ramus

The ramus of the mandible is a flat vertical plate of bone attached to the posterior part of the body.

It has inner and outer surfaces, the outer roughened by insertion of masseter muscle, the inner showing the *mandibular foramen* at about its centre. The foramen is the opening of the *mandibular canal* which transmits the *inferior alveolar nerve* and vessels and runs within the body of the bone to end near the symphysis. The terminal branches of the nerve emerge on the outer surface of the body through the mental foramen as the mental nerve.

The sharp medial lip of the foramen extends upwards and backwards as the *lingula*, to which the sphenomandibular ligament is attached. Running downwards and forwards from the foramen is the *mylohyoid groove* in which lie the mylohyoid nerve and vessels. Below and behind the groove, in the area of the angle of the jaw, is a roughening due to insertion of medial pterygoid muscle.

The upper part of the ramus consists of two processes, the *coronoid process* anteriorly and the *condylar process* posteriorly, separated by the deep *mandibular notch*. The *articular condyle* of the condylar process is supported by a narrower *neck* and articulates with the temporal bone at the temporomandibular joint. Its long axis is directed inwards and backwards.

The sharp anterior edge of the ramus runs downwards from the tip of the coronoid process to become continuous with the *external oblique line* of the body. Also, from the tip of the coronoid process, a ridge runs downwards on its inner aspect behind the third molar to become continuous with the *mylohyoid line* of the body.

The upper edge of the ramus, forming the mandibular notch, passes onto the outer side of the neck of the condyle. Medial to this ridge is the *pterygoid fovea* (fossa) on the front of the neck to which is attached the lower head of lateral pterygoid muscle.

Body

The body of the mandible is curved, and when both halves are joined they form a parabola. In its lower part it is thick and this supports the *alveolar process* which carries the lower teeth.

The outer surface of the body is fairly smooth. In the midline is a vertical ridge of bone marking the symphysis ending below in the *mental protuberance* which forms the chin. Lying on either side

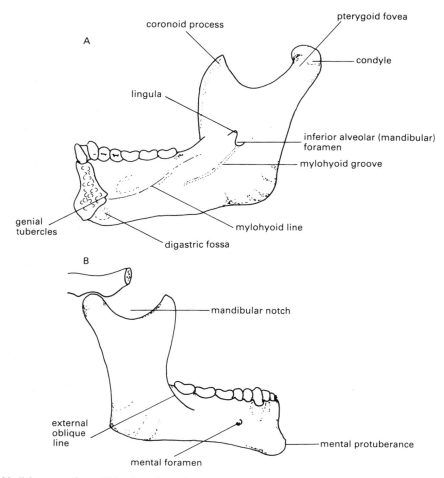

Fig. 3.2 A — Medial aspect of mandible. B — Lateral aspect.

of the midline are the paired *mental tubercles* which form part of the mental protuberance. Above, on either side of the midline below the incisor teeth, are the *incisive fossae*. Further back lies the large *mental foramen*. It is directed backwards and upwards and in the adult lies roughly midway between the lower border of the body and the upper border of the alveolar process and, although variable in position, is usually situated below the apex of the second premolar tooth.

Posterior to the foramen and passing upwards and backwards to the coronoid process is the *external oblique* line. It is more prominent posteriorly and lies between the thick basal part of the body below and the alveolar process above. To it is attached buccinator muscle. The facial artery and

vein lie on the outer surface of the bone at the anterior border of masseter muscle.

The mandible first appears on the lateral side of the inferior alveolar nerve as a band of dense mesoderm. Ossification starts in this tissue in the seventh week in the angle between the incisive and mental nerves, passes below the mental nerve, which comes to lie in a bony notch, and spreads backwards on the lateral side of the inferior alveolar nerve. The bone in the region of the notch then grows medially under the incisive nerve and then up between this nerve and Meckel's cartilage. The incisive nerve then lies in a trough of bone. Extension of bone over the mental nerve from anterior to posterior converts the notch into the mental foramen.

The trough of bone grows forward and meets its opposite partner, from which it is separated by connective tissue. Union of the two halves occurs by the end of the first postnatal year. Growth of bone over the incisive nerve converts the trough into the incisive canal. Extension of the bone in the incisor and canine region of the developing mandible engulfs Meckel's cartilage in this region and it is gradually resorbed. The most anterior part of it is taken into the bone and ossifies, possibly forming the prominent chin.

The body of the mandible from the symphysis to the mandibular foramen is produced in the foregoing fashion, and is known as the *neural element* of the bone.

Medial and *lateral alveolar plates* of bone grow upwards to form a trough above the bony incisive canal in which the developing teeth lie. This is later divided by bony septa into alveoli.

Extension backwards of the mesodermal condensation which forms the body, and subsequent ossification within this extension, forms the ramus, whose angle, coronoid and condylar processes are largely ossified by the tenth week. Further development of these processes is influenced by the development of the muscles of mastication and by the appearance of secondary cartilage. Secondary cartilage differs from primary cartilage in histological appearance and behaviour and is found in three main sites associated with the mandible.

The inner aspect of the body shows the prominent *mylohyoid line* extending from behind the last molar and passing downwards and forwards on the bone towards the midline. Mylohyoid muscle arises from this ridge. Above it, in the midline, are the *genial tubercles*, which vary in number from two pairs (an upper and a lower) to one vertical flange of bone, and give origin to the genioglossus and geniohyoid muscles.

Below the mylohyoid line near the lower border of the bone and on either side of the midline lie the small *digastric fossae* for attachment of the anterior bellies of the digastric muscles.

The sublingual and submandibular salivary glands come into contact with the inner aspect of the body. The sublingual gland lies in the *sublingual fossa* above the mylohyoid line anteriorly, the submandibular gland lies in the *submandibular fossa* below the line posteriorly.

Above the posterior part of the mylohyoid line between it and the alveolar margin and behind the third molar lies the *lingual nerve*.

The alveolar process of the mandible carries the lower teeth and is similar in many respects to the alveolar process of the maxilla. It contains sockets or *dental alveoli* for the lower teeth, the roots of which cause prominences or *alveolar juga* on its outer surface. The alveoli are separated by *interalveolar septa* and the root chambers for each tooth are separated from each other by *interradicular septa*.

The position of the teeth is not the same in the mandible as in the maxilla. The maxillary teeth form a continuous, horseshoe-shaped, curve. The lateral alveolar plate is thinner than the medial plate. In the mandible the teeth lie in a parabolic curve, the molars lying in a straight line. The lateral (labial) alveolar plate is thinner in the region of the incisors, canines and premolars but thicker than the medial (lingual) plate in the region of the molar teeth. This is accounted for by noticing that the curve of the lower arcade is sharper than the curve formed by the body of the mandible.

Since the upper and lower dental arcades have different curves they do not sit one atop the other. With the jaw closed the upper incisors lie in front of the lower ones normally, the lower incisors being directed forwards and upwards. The upper canines lie outside the lower canines and between the lower canine and first premolar teeth. The upper premolars and molars lie slightly outside the lower ones which are directed upwards and inwards so that the palatal cusps of the upper articulate between the lingual and buccal cusps of their lower counterparts. Since the upper curve is larger than the lower each upper tooth comes to articulate with its lower fellow and the tooth behind that.

Development

Each half of the mandible develops in membrane from a single centre which is formed in the first pharyngeal (mandibular) arch on the outer side of Meckel's cartilage.

Meckel's cartilage is formed earlier in fetal life and extends down from the otic capsule to meet its fellow in the midline by the sixth fetal week. It is closely related to the mandibular branch of the Vth nerve (the nerve of the arch) which divides into its lingual and inferior alveolar branches at the junction of the dorsal and middle thirds of the cartilage. The lingual nerve passes forward on the medial, and the inferior alveolar nerve on the lateral, side of the cartilage where it ends by dividing into its branches — the mental and incisive nerves.

The *condylar* cartilage appears in the twelfth week above and lateral to the bony part of the condylar process and forms a conical mass which is gradually replaced by bone by about the fifth month. However, a zone of cartilage is left beneath the articular surface of the condyle which allows for growth of the mandible and moulding of the condyle to fit the articular area on the growing temporal bone until about 20 years of age.

The *coronoid* cartilage appears slightly later along the anterior edge of the process but has gone before birth. A third area of secondary cartilage appears at the symphysis between the two halves of the mandible at about the fourteenth week. The cartilaginous masses are separated by connective tissue and fuse during the first year.

At birth the mandible differs in some respects from its adult appearance. The body of the bone has a large alveolar component full of the unerupted deciduous teeth so that the mental foramen lies close to the lower border. Once the permanent dentition is established the foramen lies halfway between the upper and lower border but in the edentulous jaw resorption of the alveolar part of the bone brings the foramen closer to the upper border where the mental nerve is then liable to pressure from an ill-fitting denture.

As the upper and lower teeth erupt the mandible must grow to accommodate them and keep them in occlusion. This is done by elongation of the body, widening of the mandible as the face widens, and elongation of the ramus. These changes alter the appearance of the mandible as it grows. At birth the angle which the ramus makes with the body is obtuse but in the adult it is almost a right-angle.

STRUCTURAL RELATIONS OF MAXILLA

The maxilla has several important structural relations. These are best appreciated by combining the examination of a dried skull, a disarticulated maxilla and radiographs, together with the palpation of bony features (in a living subject) on the face and within the oral cavity.

'Middle third of the face'

Both maxillae, together with some smaller bones (zygomatic, ethmoid, nasal and lacrimal bones), make up the middle third of the facial skeleton.

Examine the boundaries between this complex of bones and adjacent bones. Below, the maxillae are in contact with the mandible through the dental occlusion. Above, the connections are more complicated. However, the connections can be traced out if the suture between the nasal bones and the frontal bones in the midline is identified and used as a starting point. Moving laterally, identify the *frontomaxillary suture*. This is continuous with the thin suture between the *lacrimal* and *frontal* and *ethmoid* and *frontal* bones which lies just below the junction of the medial wall of the orbit and the orbital roof. About 1 cm below this line of sutures are the thin sutures between the *lacrimal* bone and *maxilla* and the *ethmoid* and *maxilla*.

Both these suture lines pass deep into the orbit and converge on a complex of sutures just below and in front of the optic foramen. The posterior aspect of the upper surface of the maxilla runs forwards and outwards marking the anterior boundary of the *inferior orbital fissure*. The *superior orbital fissure* is separated from the inferior fissure by a plate of bone which is part of the sphenoid. Near the front of the lateral wall of the orbit lie the sutures between the zygoma and the frontal bone and also between the zygoma and the sphenoid. The zygoma articulates with the maxilla in the orbit and the suture can best be identified by tracing the suture from the facial aspect into the orbit. The zygoma itself is attached via the zygomatico-temporal suture to the zygomatic process of the temporal bone, forming the zygomatic arch.

The curved posterior surface of the maxilla (viewed best from the side of the skull) is attached in its lower part to the pterygoid process of the sphenoid bone. Deep to this the maxilla articulates with the palatine bone forming part of the lateral wall of the nose and the posterior part of the bony palate.

Cavities related to the maxillary complex

The maxilla and its associated complex of small bones contributes to the major cavities of the face.

Orbit. The maxillary complex forms the orbital floor, medial wall of orbit and the zygomatic bone forms part of the lateral wall and floor of the orbital cavity.

Nasal cavity. The nasal cavity lies between both maxillae with the ethmoid above. The cribriform plate of the ethmoid separates the roof of the nasal cavity from the anterior cranial fossa.

Paranasal sinuses. The maxillary sinuses occupy the bodies of each maxilla. The other air sinuses (frontal, ethmoid and sphenoid) are extensions of the nasal cavity into the bones from which they take their names and drain their secretions into the nasal cavity.

Oral cavity. The horizontal palatal processes of the maxilla, together with the palatine bones, form the bony palate.

Alveolar bone thickness

The thickness of the buccal and palatal plates of alveolar bone determine the mode of extraction of maxillary teeth with the exception of the conically-rooted incisors. The buccal plate is relatively thinner than the palatal plate and is more deformable. Buccal movement of the maxillary teeth thereby allows the periodontal attachment to be stressed and disrupted as the buccal alveolar plate is deformed.

DENTAL EXTRACTION

General considerations

The attachment between tooth and bone is a specialised fibrous joint (periodontal membrane) which allows only limited movement. Dental extraction is the *dislocation* of the tooth/bone joint and requires that the collagen fibres of the periodontal membrane are broken.

Collagen fibres have a high tensile strength (they are thus ideally suited for transmitting masticatory forces from tooth to alveolar bone) but are relatively *inelastic* and *inextensible*. This means that if a collagen fibre is loaded and stretched its elastic limit is exceeded and the collagen fibre will break.

This basic principle forms the basis of dental extraction whereby the collagen fibres of the periodontal membrane are loaded and stretched by applying movement to the tooth by way of dental extraction forceps.

The principle is best understood by considering the extraction of a single-rooted tooth which is circular in cross-section, e.g. an upper central incisor. The tooth is gripped firmly in forceps. By attempting to *rotate* the tooth about its long axis, the collagen fibres of the periodontal membrane are loaded and stretched. As the elastic limit of the collagen is exceeded, the fibres break and the tooth can be delivered.

Only *small movements* are required to stretch the collagen fibres beyond breaking point. Where the teeth are multi-rooted, the root form precludes sizeable movements in any one direction. The necessary element of movement may be achieved by realising that the surrounding alveolar bone (when compared to the tooth) is *relatively deformable*. The tooth may be moved as a whole by deforming the alveolar bone. The direction of the movement is determined by the root form and the location of the thinner (and hence easily deformable) areas of alveolar bone. This bodily movement of the tooth loads and stretches the periodontal membrane at various sites beyond breaking point. Repeated patterns of movements will successively load, stretch and break the periodontal attachment until the tooth can be successfully delivered.

If exaggerated movements are applied, the forces generated may be enough to fracture portions of the root(s). The degree of movement necessary for extraction of teeth is gauged by clinical experience. On the whole, small controlled movements are likely to be more successful.

Extraction of maxillary teeth (Fig. 3.3)

1. *Incisors.* The conical root of a maxillary incisor can be rotated about the long axis of the tooth to sever the periodontal attachment.

2. *Canine.* The root of the maxillary canine is oval in cross-section. The large surface area of the root gives it a very strong periodontal attachment. However, the buccal plate is thin and readily deformable. The oval cross-section of the root does

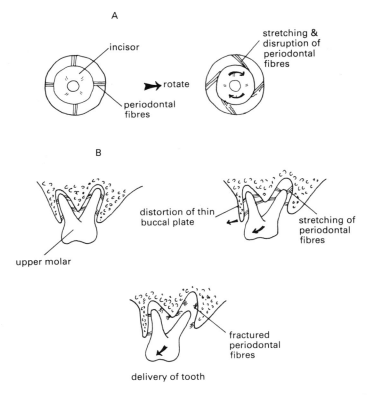

Fig. 3.3 Extraction of maxillary teeth. A — Cross-sectional view of maxillary incisor during extraction. Rotation of the tooth about its long axis stretches and fractures the fibres of the periodontal membrane. B — Extraction of an upper molar. The distortion of the thin elastic buccal bone allows the periodontal fibres to be stretched and fractured.

allow slight to-and-fro rotatory movements and this, together with movement to deform the buccal plate, is sufficient to disrupt its strong attachment.

3. *Premolars.* The first premolar tooth may have two roots (buccal and palatal), of which the buccal tends to be the thinner and liable to fracture during extraction. The buccal plate of bone is thin and deformable and the predominant movement in the extraction is, therefore, buccal.

The second premolar tooth has a single root, oval in cross-section. The same considerations that are pertinent to the maxillary canine may be applied but the surface area of the root is much less and the periodontal attachment is not as strong.

4. *Molars.* The two buccal and one palatal roots of the maxillary molar teeth preclude any rotation of these teeth about their long axis during extraction. The buccal plate is thin, especially related to the third molar, but can be thick over the first molar, particularly if the zygomatic process of the

maxilla arises low down. In any event the buccal plate is more deformable than the palatal plate and these teeth can be extracted by deforming or expanding the socket by applying a downwards and buccal movement to the tooth.

Variation in root form and number

Variation in the *number, size* and *orientation* of roots is common, particularly third molars. The orientation of roots may also vary, for example, when teeth have rotated from their normal position. *These variations are best detected by the examination of good radiographs*, such as the intraoral periapical view.

Extraction of maxillary third molars

Partially and fully erupted upper third molars are frequently orientated with the crown facing buccally and backwards. Access to such teeth with forceps is restricted, not only by their unfavourable inclination, but also by the coronoid process of the mandible moving forwards to lie above and lateral to the maxillary tuberosity when the mouth is opened. Where this occurs the teeth may be extracted using elevators if the root form is favourable. Extreme care is required as the tooth may be displaced backwards into the deep tissues of the infratemporal fossa.

Unerupted third molar teeth require surgical extraction. Depending on their orientation and degree of eruption, they can lie at variable positions on the maxillary tuberosity and closely related to the maxillary air sinus. Posterior displacement of the tooth into the infratemporal fossa or upwards displacement into the maxillary air sinus can result from careless use of elevators.

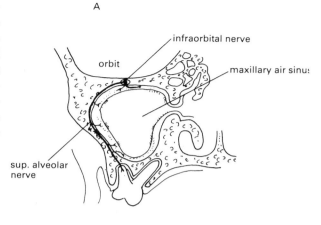

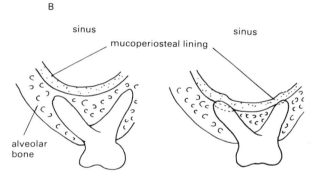

Relationship between maxillary teeth and the maxillary air sinus (Fig. 3.4)

The root apices of the second premolar and the three molar teeth are intimately related to the maxillary air sinus. The relationship is variable; the apices of some or all of these teeth may be separated from the mucous membrane by a thin layer of bone and in some instances may only be separated from the sinus cavity by the mucous membrane itself. In either event the close proximity of the sinus may lead to complications following dental extraction.

Oroantral fistula. A fistula connecting the oral cavity with the maxillary air sinus may be established during extraction of the maxillary second premolar or the molar teeth. If suspected, it can be confirmed immediately after extraction by asking the patient to occlude the nostrils and to attempt to breathe out through the nose. The increased air pressure in the nasal cavity will force air to bubble through the fistula forming 'bloody bubbles'. Occasionally, however, if the antral mucosa is intact, the mucosa may bulge down into the extraction socket. It has a bluish tinge due to the presence of mucous glands.

The formation of a firm postextraction clot will seal off most small oroantral fistulas, which then heal. Patients should be instructed to avoid sneezing (causing large increases in intrasinus air press-

Fig. 3.4 A — Coronal section of maxillary sinus. The sinus floor lies at a lower level than the floor of the nasal cavity. B — The relationship of maxillary teeth to the sinus.

ure) which might prejudice successful closure of the fistula.

Chronic oroantral fistula. The persistence of a fistula can have unpleasant consequences. Oral micro-organisms enter the sinus and give rise to a *maxillary sinusitis.* During swallowing of liquids and foodstuffs, some may be forced through the fistula to enter the sinus and eventually emerge from the nostril and back of the nose.

Chronic fistulas require surgical repair by removing the fistula track and covering the defect with an 'advancement' flap of buccal or palatal mucosa.

Displacement of root fragments into the maxillary air sinus

Fractures of the roots of second premolar and molar maxillary teeth can occur during attempted extraction despite careful technique. Attempts to remove the fragments by the application of elevators may displace the root fragment upwards into the maxillary air sinus. This leads to maxillary sinusitis and the root fragment can only be removed surgically.

Fractures of the maxillary tuberosity

The maxilla is able to withstand *vertical* loading forces due to mastication. Dental extraction involves the application of sizeable *horizontal* forces to the alveolar process of the maxilla and this may cause small portions of the buccal alveolar plate to fracture during extraction. The distal part of the alveolar process of the maxilla, i.e. the maxillary tuberosity and the alveolar bone forming the socket of the third molar, is particularly susceptible to fracture particularly if the third molar is lone standing.

Fractures of the maxillary tuberosity require minor surgical intervention to remove the bony fragments and careful closure of the wound edges to seal off the invariable oroantral fistula.

MAXILLARY AIR SINUS (Fig. 3.4)

The body of the maxilla is occupied by an air sinus which is *pyramidal* in shape. The base is formed by the lateral wall of the nose and the apex extends into the zygomatic process of the maxilla and in some instances even extends further into the body of the zygomatic bone.

The roof of the air sinus forms the thin bony floor of the orbital cavity. A ridge, raised by the infraorbital canal, runs forwards across the roof of the air sinus. The anterior superior alveolar and middle superior alveolar nerves run in bony canals from the infraorbital canal down the lateral wall of the sinus and also give rise to bony ridges.

The floor of the maxillary air sinus is closely related to the maxillary teeth. Ridges of bone corresponding to the alveolar septa of the underlying teeth are found. In some instances the apices of the molar teeth may project through the bone into the sinus where they are only covered by mucous membrane.

The floor of the sinus lies about 1.25 cm *below* the level of the nasal floor. The sinus drains from an opening through its medial wall into the middle meatus of the nose.

The mucous membrane lining the sinus is a mucoperiosteum. The epithelium is respiratory in type. The mucus produced by the goblet cells is directed by ciliary action toward the sinus opening to drain into the nasal cavity. Since the opening lies nearer the roof of the sinus than its floor, overproduction of mucus results in its 'pooling' under gravity in the sinus.

The sensory nerve supply of the mucous membrane is derived from adjacent nerves; the infraorbital nerve and the posterior, middle and anterior superior alveolar nerves. The lymphatic drainage is to the submandibular lymph nodes.

Clinical considerations
Examination of maxillary sinuses

Transillumination. If an electric torch is placed in the mouth in a darkened room a red glow is observed on the face in the region of the sinus. In a diseased or fluid-filled sinus this effect will be absent due to the absorbtion of the light by the sinus contents.

Radiographic examination. Normal sinuses are radiolucent. The presence of fluid in a diseased sinus renders it radio-opaque. The presence of fluid and the extent to which the sinus is filled is readily seen in anteroposterior radiographs. Lateral radiographs reveal the proximity of the roots of the maxillary molar teeth to the sinus floor.

Sinusitis

Viral infections of the upper respiratory tract occur frequently, e.g. the common cold.

In *acute sinusitis* the mucous membrane of the sinus produces large amounts of secretions which are not drained away. A feeling of pressure and tension in the sinus results.

Secondary bacterial infection of a congested sinus results in an *acute suppurative sinusitis*. The presence of pus under pressure results in pain over the sinus and eye. The maxillary molar teeth may be tender to percussion.

In *chronic sinusitis* one or more of the maxillary sinuses remains infected with a pyogenic organism. Loss of cilia from the mucosa can occur in longstanding chronic infections. This obviously impairs the drainage of the sinus and episodes of acute sinusitis are more likely to recur.

Infections of dental origin

The proximity of the maxillary molar teeth to the maxillary sinus may result in the spread of infection from the teeth to the maxillary sinus, resulting in an acute sinusitis.

Referred pain

Since the maxillary teeth and supporting tissues and the maxillary sinus receive their sensory nerve supply from the superior alveolar nerves, the phenomenon of referred pain can result in disease originating in the sinus manifesting itself as pain associated with maxillary teeth and vice versa.

Where no dental cause can be found to explain the symptoms, it is necessary to then examine the maxillary sinuses.

Tumours of the maxillary sinus

Malignant tumours arising from the mucosa of the maxillary sinus may invade the supporting bone of the molar teeth rendering them mobile. Pressure exerted by the growing lesion on the superior alveolar nerves and on the infraorbital nerves can cause parasthesia in the tissues supplied by these nerves, teeth, mucous membrane of gingiva and cheek and the skin in the area of distribution of the infraorbital nerve.

Maxillary fractures

Fractures of the middle third of the face

The bones of the middle third of the facial skeleton can withstand very high masticatory loads acting vertically. Forces acting in a horizontal direction tend to displace the middle third of the facial skeleton *posteriorly*. In effect, the bony complex is sheared off relative to the extremely robust bones of the vault.

Dentoalveolar fractures

Fractures of isolated segments of alveolar bone containing one or more teeth can occur. Fractures of the tuberosity are described elsewhere and are a common type of dentoalveolar fracture.

Le Fort type fractures (Fig. 3.5)

Experiments carried out by le Fort in which the heads of cadavers were subjected to various degrees of trauma indicated that fractures of the middle third of the facial skeleton tended to occur in three broad categories.

In le Fort type 1 fractures the fracture involves the lower part of the maxilla, lateral nasal wall and lower part of the pterygoid plates of the sphenoid.

In le Fort type 2 fractures the central portion of the maxilla is fractured from the rest of the facial skeleton.

In le Fort type 3 fractures the entire middle third of the facial skeleton is involved. Posterior displacement occurs relative to the base of the skull.

Signs and symptoms of maxillary fracture

These depend on the severity of the injury, the way the injury was sustained and the type of fracture (le Fort). Since the middle third of the facial skeleton contains the major cavities of the face, damage to these and the structures therein may produce associated signs and symptoms.

Oedema of the soft tissues over the middle third of the face is characteristically severe.

Haemorrhage into the tissues around the eye (circumorbital ecchymosis) and into the subconjunctival tissues (subconjunctival ecchymosis) when the orbital floor or wall is damaged (le Fort 2 and 3 type injuries).

Posterior displacement of the maxilla. The displacement of the maxilla against the sloping cranial base tends to 'lengthen the face' by forcing the mandible open due to gagging of the occlusion in the molar region. A 'dish face' is also present, in skeletal terms, but is masked by the massive oedema of the facial tissues.

Intraorally. Gagging of the occlusion occurs and damage to the superior alveolar nerves may cause anaesthesia of the teeth.

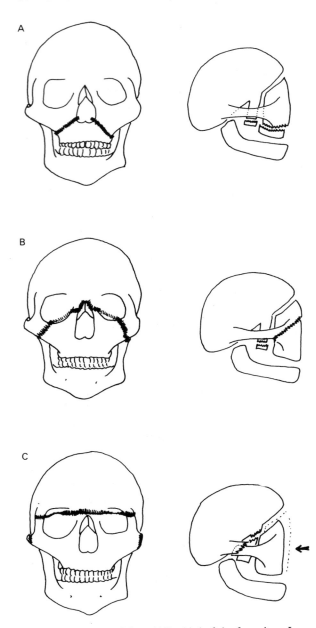

Fig. 3.5 Fractures of the middle third of the face. A — Le Fort 1. B — Le Fort 2. C — Le Fort 3.

Percussion of the maxillary teeth where the maxilla is fractured produces a sound akin to the striking of a 'cracked tea-cup'.

Midline separation of the maxilla can occur in middle third fractures allowing the oral cavity to communicate with the nasal cavity.

Treatment of fractures of the middle third of the face

Middle third fractures are treated by:
1. *Reduction of displaced bone ends.*
2. *Immobilisation of fragments* to allow fracture repair.
3. *Control of infection.*

Since the middle third of the facial skeleton is so complex the reduction and immobilisation of the many fractures that occur within this bony complex is extremely complicated. Severe injuries may, when the bony complex has been displaced posteriorly, require disimpaction and the treatment of associated injuries to the cranial, orbital and nasal cavities. Immobilisation of the bony segments is achieved by wiring the fragments together and attaching these to splints, the mandible (if unaffected) or the intact cranium.

STRUCTURAL RELATIONS OF MANDIBLE (Fig. 3.6)

Inferior alveolar nerve

This nerve descends through the infratemporal fossa and enters the mandibular foramen, after passing between the mandibular ramus and the sphenomandibular ligament, to run forward through the mandible in the inferior alveolar canal. Studies have suggested that the situation may be more complicated. The nerve may branch before reaching the mandible and these small accessory branches then enter the mandible through small and inconstant foramina on the mandibular ramus. In addition, sensory branches from the associated mandibular muscles or the buccal nerve also enter the mandible. The main nerve bundle and these accessory branches form a complicated nerve plexus in the mandible. Thus, individual teeth may receive their nerve supply from:
1. Inferior alveolar nerve (mandibular foramen).
2. Accessory branches (accessory foramina on ramus).
3. Sensory nerves coming from muscles (e.g. masseter).

The main inferior alveolar nerve, together with an associated artery and vein, runs through the mandible in a well-defined bony canal. The in-

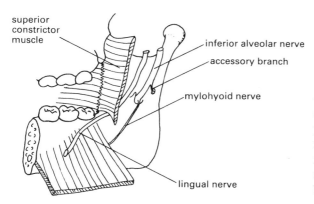

superior constrictor muscle

inferior alveolar nerve

accessory branch

mylohyoid nerve

lingual nerve

Fig. 3.6 The inferior alveolar and lingual nerves.

ferior alveolar canal lies below the apices of the teeth. The proximity of the canal to the roots of the teeth varies. In unerupted teeth, particularly third molars, the inferior neurovascular bundle may be in *contact* with or even *perforate* the roots of the third molar tooth.

Lingual nerve

The lingual nerve approaches the mandible by passing downwards and forwards between the ramus and medial pterygoid muscle. It passes below the mandibular origin of the superior constrictor muscle. At this point it lies *in contact with the mandible* on the medial aspect of the lingual alveolus of the third molar. Since it is only covered by mucous membrane at this point, the lingual nerve can be palpated readily. It then sweeps forwards away from the mandible to the side of the tongue.

Mental nerve

This branches from the inferior alveolar nerve and emerges from the mandible through the mental foramen to supply adjacent mucous membrane and skin of the lower lip.

Clinical considerations

1. Inferior alveolar local anaesthesia: local anaesthesia of the structures supplied by this nerve is obtained by depositing anaesthetic solution around the nerve as it enters the mandibular foramen. The existence of sensory nerve fibres entering the mandible at other sites may account for the failure to achieve complete anaesthesia.

2. Relationship between inferior alveolar nerve and third molar teeth: the position of the inferior alveolar nerve relative to a partially erupted or impacted third molar tooth must be determined before these teeth are removed. This can be done radiographically. Damage to the nerve would result in a loss of sensation in the tissues supplied by the nerve.

3. Lingual nerve: the close proximity of the lingual nerve to the rim of the socket of the third molar tooth renders it liable to trauma during the removal of these teeth whether by forceps or surgical extraction.

4. Mental nerve: in minor surgical procedures in the premolar region, care must be taken to avoid damage to the mental nerve.

Alveolar bone thickness

As with the maxilla, the thickness of the mandibular alveolar bone determines the mode of extraction of mandibular teeth. Unlike the maxilla, the relative thickness of the outer alveolar and inner alveolar bony walls shows considerable variation in the mandible. The labial alveolar bone related to the incisors and canines is thinner and hence more deformable than the lingual. As one moves progressively from the premolar teeth, where the lingual and buccal plates are similar in thickness, to the third molar tooth, the buccal bone increases in thickness and the lingual bone decreases, but not to such a marked extent.

Clinical considerations

Extraction of mandibular teeth (Fig. 3.7)

Incisors. The short roots of mandibular incisors are oval in cross-section. Rotation of these teeth is not possible. The thin, deformable labial alveolar bone allows the teeth to be displaced buccally so severing the periodontal attachment.

Canine. The mandibular canine has a long root, oval in cross-section. Its large root surface area

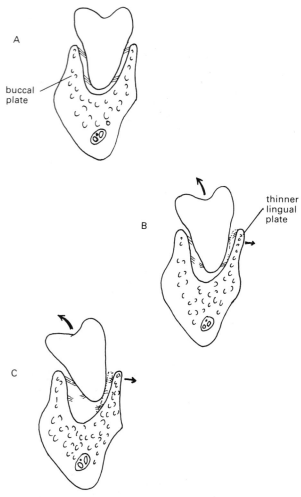

buccal
plate

A

thinner
lingual
plate

B

C

Fig. 3.7 Extraction of mandibular molars. Distortion of the lingual bony plate allows the periodontal fibres to be stretched and fractured.

gives it a strong attachment. As with the incisor teeth, the labial alveolar plate is deformable and allows the periodontal attachment to be severed using a combination of movements in which the buccal direction predominates.

Premolars. The single roots of the premolar teeth are circular in cross-section. While usually straight, they occasionally show a slight distal curve towards the apex. Rotation about the long axis is sufficient to disrupt the periodontal attachment.

Molars. The mandibular molar teeth have two sturdy roots — mesial and distal — which usually have a slight distal curvature. Each root is ellip-

soidal in cross-section, the long axis of the ellipse lying buccolingually. Since the lingual alveolar plate is thinner and more deformable than the buccal plate, the periodontal attachment can be severed by displacing the tooth upwards and buccally so that the lingual plate is deformed (Fig. 3.7). The roots being thickest buccolingually are strong enough to withstand the high forces involved.

The position of the mandibular third molar tooth at the back of the dental arch may sometimes hinder the correct positioning of extraction forceps.

Variation in root form and number

Variation in the *number*, *size* and *orientation* of roots is common, particularly third molars. *These variations are best detected by the examination of good radiographs.*

Impacted mandibular third molar teeth (Fig. 3.8)

The third molar teeth are the last to erupt. If insufficient room exists in the dental arch, the normal eruption of the tooth may be frustrated and the tooth becomes *impacted* or *displaced* from its optimum position in the dental arch. This is a common occurrence. Mandibular third molar teeth are usually removed since;

1. They are *impacted* and look like remaining so.
2. They are causing *pain* and *discomfort* for the patient.
3. The soft tissues around the crown of partially erupted mandibular third molars are especially susceptible to infection (pericoronitis).

The mandible is at its thickest in the region of the third molar. Extraction of abnormally positioned third molars usually involves the removal of bone around the tooth to relieve the impaction (Fig. 3.8).

The *position* of the tooth relative to the surrounding bony landmarks is one of the main determinants in the preoperative assessment of the degree of difficulty of the extraction. This can be determined by palpation of the retromolar area and examination of radiographs. The intraoral periapical view is especially valuable in defining the pos-

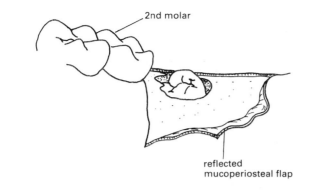

2nd molar

reflected
mucoperiosteal flap

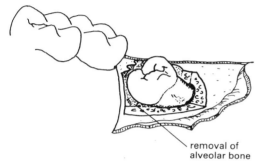

removal of
alveolar bone

Fig. 3.8 Impacted third molars require alveolar bone to be removed during their extraction. This in itself can weaken the mandible.

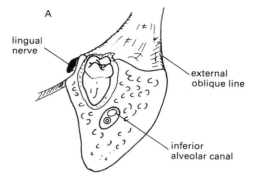

A

lingual nerve

external oblique line

inferior alveolar canal

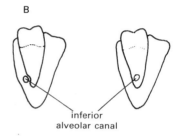

B

inferior alveolar canal

Fig. 3.9 A — Coronal section of mandible just in front of the third molar. Note the proximity of the lingual nerve to the crest of the alveolus. B — The roots of unerupted third molars may be grooved or even pierced by the inferior alveolar neurovascular bundle.

ition and angulation of the tooth and the configuration and number of its roots (Fig. 3.9).

Mandibular fractures

Although a robust bone, the mandible is liable to fracture following intentional or unintentional violence. Fractures tend to occur at specific sites depending on the nature of the violence. These are (Fig. 3.10):

1. Condylar head.
2. Ramus.
3. Angle of mandible.
4. Body of mandible.

The nature and severity of the injury will depend on whether the fracture is unilateral or multiple and whether tissue loss is present. The muscles acting on the mandible may also influence the degree of displacement at the fracture site, depending on the orientation of the line of fracture (Fig. 3.10).

Condylar head fractures

The condyle lies within the capsule of the TMJ. Fractures of the condylar head may occur within the capsule or more commonly be extracapsular. In both instances, the lateral pterygoid muscle which is attached to the condylar head tends to displace the condylar head forwards out of the glenoid fossa.

Fractures of the ramus

Displacement of the fractured segments is minimal as the fragments tend to be splinted together between the masseter and medial pterygoid muscles.

Fractures of the angle and body

Fractures of the angle and body are invariably *compound* due to the presence of teeth and allow micro-organisms entry to the fracture site. The

A

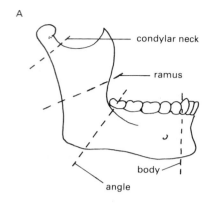

condylar neck

ramus

body

angle

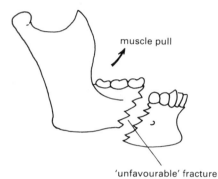

muscle pull

'unfavourable' fracture

B

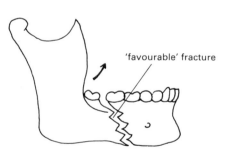

'favourable' fracture

C

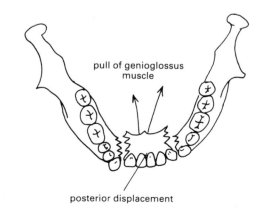

pull of genioglossus
muscle

posterior displacement

presence of unerupted teeth, particularly the third molar, 'weakens' the mandible and predisposes towards fracture at that site. Similarly, the long root of the canine constitutes a 'weak spot' and fractures in that region are common.

The *inferior alveolar neurovascular bundle* is damaged in fractures of the mandibular body. The degree of damage depends on the displacement of the bone ends and can vary from traumatic stretching of the bundle to complete severance. Damage to the inferior alveolar artery is not critical since the mandible receives an adequate collateral blood supply. Damage to the inferior alveolar nerve will result in loss or reduction of sensation in the area supplied by the nerve. If the fracture is treated successfully the repair process may be sufficient to restore full sensation but partial anaesthesia or parasthesia may persist.

Bilateral fractures of the mandible (Fig. 3.10)

Bilateral fractures of the anterior body of the mandible are especially important since the segment of bone to which genioglossus muscle is attached may be displaced posteriorly. Since genioglossus is the *only* muscle which acts to maintain the tongue in a forward position, the loss of its skeletal anchorage will result in the tongue being displaced *posteriorly* with resulting respiratory embarrassment.

Fractures of the glenoid fossa

Mandibular trauma and especially condylar head fractures may involve the impaction of the condylar head through the glenoid fossa into the middle cranial fossa. The middle ear cavity and external auditory meatus will be involved and haemorrhage from the external ear will occur.

Signs and symptoms of mandibular fractures

History of injury

Pain is present, associated with movement of the jaw.

Fig. 3.10 A — Common sites of mandibular fractures. B — The powerful muscles acting on the mandible can affect displacement of the fracture segments. C — Bilateral fractures in the anterior body of the mandible can cause the tongue to fall backwards and jeopardise the airway.

Reduced mobility and *abnormal function*, e.g. during mastication. The extent to which these occur depends upon the extent of the injury and the degree of displacement of the bony segments. Such displacement may be *minimal*, such as in some fractures of the condyle.

Malocclusion of the teeth is present if there has been displacement of the bony segments. Malocclusions can also be found in jaws which have not been fractured.

Swelling of the soft tissues related to the fracture site is found and since the fractures involve damage to periosteum, which is a highly vascular tissue, this will be accompanied by bruising.

In fractures of the body of the mandible periosteal bleeding at the fracture site occurs into the *buccal sulcus* and *sublingual space*. A *sub-lingual haematoma* is a classic sign of mandibular fracture.

Treatment of mandibular fractures

Mandibular fractures are treated by:
1. *Reduction of the displaced bone ends.*
2. *Immobilisation of the fragments* to allow fracture repair to be effected.
3. *Control of infection* to allow fracture repair to be successful.

Mandibular fractures can be immobilised using a variety of methods such as wiring the fragments together and fixing this to splints, the maxillary teeth or stabilising bars. Alternatively, the bone ends can be wired together directly or fixed using alloy plates.

4

Neurology

CRANIAL NERVES

The 12 pairs of cranial nerves are part of the peripheral nervous system and emerge from the base of the brain. Each nerve is named and also bears a Roman numeral, by convention. Details of each nerve are set out below.

Cranial nerve I (olfactory)

The special sense of smell is mediated by this nerve. Peripheral processes of bipolar olfactory cells lie within the nasal mucosa of the roof, the superior concha and the upper part of the septum of the nasal cavity. Their central processes pass through the *cribriform plate* into the anterior cranial fossa as 15 to 20 branches and synapse in the mitral cells of the olfactory *bulbs* which lie on the intracranial aspect of the cribriform plate.

The central processes of the mitral cells pass back in the olfactory *tract* to the olfactory area of the cortex, the paraterminal gyrus and prepiriform cortex.

Clinical considerations

Anosmia, loss of the sense of smell, may be unilateral or bilateral. Bilateral anosmia is commonly caused by colds and other forms of rhinitis but may also be due to olfactory nerve involvement in fractures of the anterior cranial fossa and may be associated in this case with c.s.f. rhinorrhea. Unilateral anosmia may be symptomatic of frontal lobe tumours involving one of the olfactory nerves. Tumours involving the olfactory area of the cortex may give rise to olfactory hallucinations.

Clinical testing of the olfactory nerve. Each nostril is tested separately using bottles of common test odours. Identification or even awareness of the odour precludes anosmia of that side.

Cranial nerve II (optic)

The special sense of sight is mediated by the optic nerve. Light passing into the eyeball is focused onto the retina whose cells are arranged into three layers.

The deepest retinal layer consists of the *rods* and *cones*, which are photoreceptor cells, the rods being sensitive to low intensity light and movement and the cones to high intensity light and colour. Their processes pass superficially to an intermediate layer of *bipolar cells* and their processes, in turn, pass to the superficial layer of *ganglion* cells whose processes pass to the optic disc and leave the eyeball as the *optic nerve*.

The optic nerve leaves the orbit through the optic canal and joins its fellow of the opposite side at the optic *chiasma*. Here, the fibres from the nasal half of each retina decussate (the fibres from the temporal halves remaining uncrossed), join the temporal fibres from the opposite retina, and form the optic *tract*.

Fibres of the optic tract pass to (1) the lateral geniculate body and (2) the superior colliculus and the pretectal area.

1. Cells within the lateral geniculate body send fibres, the *optic radiations*, to that part of the occipital cortex which lies around the *calcarine sulcus*, those ending above the sulcus relay impulses from the lower parts of the visual fields, those ending below the sulcus from the upper parts of the visual fields.

2. Fibres from this area pass to the *Edinger-*

Westphal nucleus of the midbrain whose axons pass via the oculomotor nerve and the ciliary ganglion to the sphincter pupillae. These facilitate the direct and consensual light reflexes.

Fibres also pass to other cranial nuclei to facilitate other ocular reflexes, e.g. involuntary protective reflexes.

Clinical considerations

Many conditions may affect or involve the eye and the visual pathway and only a few examples are mentioned below to illustrate the effects of interruption of the pathway at various sites.

1. Lesions involving the retina or the optic nerve of one side result in unilateral symptoms. Complete destruction will cause unilateral blindness; partial involvement will cause a loss of vision in the affected areas (scotoma).

2. Bilateral involvement of the eyes may be due to generalised disorders, e.g. hypertension, diabetes, multiple sclerosis.

3. Lesions of the chiasma, e.g. by compression from an expanding pituitary tumour, will disrupt the fibres from the nasal halves of both retinae as they decussate and give rise to temporal field defects in each eye, *bitemporal hemianopia.*

4. Lesions to one side of the chiasma, e.g. internal carotid artery aneurysm, may produce a *unilateral nasal hemianopia* by involving fibres from the temporal half on one retina only.

5. Lesions of the optic tract disrupt the fibres from the ipsilateral sides of both retinae and result in *homonymous hemianopia* with pupillary involvement (loss of light reflexes).

6. Lesions of the optic radiations also result in homonymous field defects but with preservation of the light reflexes. Lesions which involve the occipital cortex *above* the calcarine sulcus produce homonymous *inferior quadrant* defects, those below the sulcus homonymous *superior quadrant* defects.

Clinical testing of the optic nerve. Testing is divided into the following categories:

1. Visual *acuity* is tested using standard card tests.

2. Visual *fields* are tested by using simple confrontation tests which compare the examinees visual fields with the examiners. Visual field mapping can be carried out by perimetry.

3. Colour perception can be tested by standard cards.

4. The retina, optic disc and vessels and other intraocular structures can be directly visualised by the use of ophthalmoscope or slit-lamp.

Cranial nerve III (oculomotor)

The third, fourth and sixth cranial nerves are all motor nerves to the extraocular muscles and are dealt with below. The sixth nerve, therefore, appears out of sequence.

The third nerve is a motor nerve supplying most of the extraocular muscles of the eyeball and the levator palpebrae superioris muscle of the upper eyelid. It also transmits *preganglionic parasympathetic* fibres to the *ciliary ganglion.*

The motor fibres of the third nerve arise from a group of nuclei in the midbrain, the *oculomotor nucleus*, and emerge from the brain stem in the interpeduncular fossa between the cerebral peduncles, some fibres passing through the red nucleus and the medial part of the peduncle en route. The nerve passes forwards, closely related to the edge of the tentorium cerebelli, pierces the dura to run in the lateral wall of the cavernous sinus, divides into superior and inferior branches and enters the orbit through the superior orbital fissure. The *superior* branch supplies superior rectus and levator palpebrae superioris muscles and the *inferior* branch supplies medial rectus, inferior rectus and inferior oblique muscles, the nerve to inferior oblique giving off a branch to the ciliary ganglion.

Preganglionic parasympathetic fibres arise from the *Edinger-Westphal nucleus* of the midbrain and run with the oculomotor nerve to the ciliary ganglion, lateral to the optic nerve, where they synapse. *Post-ganglionic* fibres run via *short ciliary nerves* to the ciliary and sphincter pupillae muscles.

Clinical considerations

Lesions, e.g. tumour, haemorrhage, aneurysm of the circle of Willis, which completely paralyse the oculomotor nerve give rise to the following signs and symptoms.

1. *Pupillary dilatation* (mydriasis): due to the unopposed action of sympathetic fibres on the pupillary muscles.

2. *Divergent strabismus* (external squint): due to paralysis of the extraocular muscles supplied by the oculomotor nerve. The affected eye is deviated outwardly and loses the ability to rotate inwardly.

3. *Diplopia* (double vision): since the eyes will not move synchronously in certain directions a double image is perceived.

4. *Ptosis* (drooping of upper eyelid): due to paralysis of levator palpebrae superioris.

5. *Loss of light and accommodation reflexes*: since both the sphincter pupillae and ciliary muscles are paralysed.

Increasing intracranial pressure due to a rapidly growing tumour or haemorrhage following trauma and skull fracture may manifest itself first as pupillary dilatation due to compression of the oculomotor nerve against the edge of the tentorium cerebelli. Incomplete lesions of the third nerve may produce a slight weakness in all of its functions or one symptom alone may be present.

Clinical testing of the oculomotor nerve. The motor and parasympathetic components of oculomotor nerve function are tested using:

1. Finger-following tests, in which the examinee is instructed to follow the examiner's finger with his eyes in all the cardinal directions of gaze, to determine whether there is a paralysis of one or more of the extraocular muscles. The presence and direction of diplopia can be roughly detected in this fashion also.

2. A pocket-torch, shone onto the eye from the side to eliminate an accommodation reflex, will demonstrate the presence or absence of direct and consensual light reflexes. Remember that this test depends upon the integrity of the optic nerve also. The accommodation reflex is tested by asking the patient to focus upon an object approaching him.

Cranial nerve IV (trochlear)

The trochlear nerve is the motor nerve to the superior oblique muscle of the eyeball. Its fibres arise from the *trochlear nucleus*, situated below the oculomotor nucleus in the region of the inferior colliculus of the midbrain, and pass dorsally, decussating in the anterior medullary velum, to emerge from the *dorsum* of the brain stem. The nerve then winds around the cerebral peduncle and comes to lie lateral to the third nerve which it follows through the cavernous sinus and the superior orbital fissure into the orbit.

Clinical considerations

Isolated lesions of the trochlear nerve are uncommon and will result in diplopia on gaze downward and laterally. First indications of a lesion of this nature may arise by experiencing diplopia during reading or descending stairs.

Clinical testing of the trochlear nerve. The presence of paralysis and diplopia can be detected by finger-following tests as for III (above).

Cranial nerve VI (abducens)

The abducens nerve, like the trochlear, is a motor nerve to one extraocular muscle. In this case, the lateral rectus muscle. Its fibres arise from the *abducens nucleus*, which lies in the pons below the fourth ventricle, and leave the brain stem anteriorly between the pons and the medulla. The nerve runs in a long course through the posterior cranial fossa, over the apex of the petrous temporal bone, and enters the cavernous sinus, which it traverses in close relation to the internal carotid artery. It passes into the orbit through the superior orbital fissure.

Clinical considerations

Sixth nerve palsy is the commonest of eye palsies since the nerve has such a long course within the skull. Fractures of the skull base or increasing intracranial pressure may affect the nerve giving rise to an *internal strabismus* and *diplopia* on outward gaze. The patient may turn his head to the affected side to alleviate this.

Clinical testing of the abducens nerve. The presence of paralysis and diplopia can be detected by finger-following tests as for III and IV (above).

The optic nerves, which mediate our sense of sight, and the nuclei of the three nerves which control movements of the eyes are interconnected by tract systems which are involved in certain eye reflexes. The light and accommodation reflexes have been discussed but the third, fourth and sixth nuclei and the visual pathway also mediate eye reflexes connected with hearing and balance, fixation reflexes and protective reflexes which act to close the eyes (via VIIth nerve) or involve the limb and body musculature (via tectospinal fibres).

Cranial nerve V (trigeminal)

The trigeminal nerve consists of a large *sensory root*, which supplies much of the skin and mucous membrane of the head, and a smaller *motor root*, which supplies the muscles of mastication.

Both components emerge from the pons onto the petrous temporal bone near its apex. Here the nerve flattens out into the *trigeminal ganglion*, which lies in a bony depression. The three *divisions* of the nerve, the *ophthalmic, maxillary* and *mandibular* divisions arise from the ganglion, the motor root travelling with the mandibular division.

Distribution of Divisions

1. *Ophthalmic*. The ophthalmic nerve passes forwards into the lateral wall of the cavernous sinus and divides into three branches, the *frontal, lacrimal*, and *nasociliary* nerves, which enter the orbit through the superior orbital fissure.

The frontal nerve runs below the roof of the orbit and divides into *supraorbital* and *supratrochlear* branches. The supraorbital nerve passes through the supraorbital foramen or notch and runs upwards to supply the skin of the forehead and scalp as far as the vertex, and the mucous membrane of the frontal sinus. The supratrochlear nerve leaves the upper medial angle of the orbit to supply the upper eyelid and the forehead above the nose.

The lacrimal nerve runs along the lateral wall of the orbit, receives *post-ganglionic parasympathetic secretomotor* fibres (from the sphenopalatine ganglion via the zygomatic branch of the maxillary nerve) with which it supplies the lacrimal gland, and supplies the skin and conjunctiva of the lateral part of the upper eyelid.

The nasociliary nerve runs along the medial wall of the orbit and gives branches to the *ciliary ganglion* and branches, the *long ciliary nerves*, directly to the eyeball. Sympathetic fibres from the internal carotid plexus pass with the long ciliary nerves to the dilator pupillae muscle. Other branches of the nasociliary nerve are:

1. The *posterior ethmoidal* nerve which supplies the sphenoidal and posterior ethmoidal air cells.

2. The *anterior ethmoidal* nerve which passes through the foramen of the same name to enter and supply the dura of the anterior cranial fossa, descends into the nasal cavity through the cribriform plate to supply the mucous membrane of the upper part of the nasal cavity, and emerges between the nasal bone and cartilage as the *external nasal* nerve to supply an area of skin over the nose.

3. The *infratrochlear* nerve which leaves the orbit medially and supplies the skin and conjunctiva at the medial angle of the eye, skin of the adjacent part of the nose and the lacrimal sac and duct.

2. *Maxillary*. The maxillary nerve runs forwards from the trigeminal ganglion and passes through the *foramen rotundum* to enter the pterygopalatine fossa, where the *pterygopalatine ganglion* is suspended from the nerve, and where it gives off the following branches.

The *zygomatic* nerve enters the orbit through the inferior orbital fissure and carries parasympathetic fibres from the pterygopalatine ganglion to join the lacrimal nerve. Its terminal branches are the *zygomaticotemporal* and *zygomaticofacial* nerves which emerge from the zygomatic bone to supply the skin of the temple and malar area, respectively.

The *posterior superior alveolar* nerve runs downwards on the infratemporal surface of the maxilla, divides into three or four branches, and enters small foramina on the posterior aspect of the maxilla to run forward and supply the mucosa of the maxillary sinus and the upper molar teeth (except the mesiobuccal root of the first molar). Small branches which do not enter the bone supply the buccal gum of these teeth.

Ganglionic branches pass to the pterygopalatine ganglion which therefore receives *sensory* fibres from the maxillary nerve as well as postganglionic *sympathetic* fibres from the internal carotid plexus via the *deep petrosal* nerve and *preganglionic parasympathetic* fibres from the geniculate ganglion of the VIIth nerve via the *greater superficial petrosal* nerve. The parasympathetic fibres synapse in the ganglion. Nerves arising from the pterygopalatine ganglion contain fibres of all three types and are distributed as follows.

The *greater palatine* nerve runs downwards to emerge onto the hard palate through the greater palatine foramen. It runs forwards along the hard palate in the angle between the alveolar and palatal processes to supply the mucous membrane and glands of the hard palate, except for the triangular incisive area behind the anterior teeth, and the palatal gum.

The *lesser palatine* nerves run with the greater palatine nerves to emerge through the lesser palatine foramina and supply glands and mucous membrane of the soft palate.

The *nasopalatine* (long sphenopalatine) nerve passes medially through the sphenopalatine foramen, across the roof of the nasal cavity, and then downwards on the nasal septum, supplying the septal mucosa, to enter the incisive canal and supply the mucous membrane and gum of the incisive area. *Nasal* (short sphenopalatine nerves) and *pharyngeal* branches run with the nasopalatine nerve through the sphenopalatine foramen to supply the lateral wall of the nasal cavity and the pharyngeal roof, respectively.

The terminal portion of the maxillary nerve passes through the inferior orbital fissure and enters the *infraorbital groove* as the *infraorbital* nerve. This runs forwards into the *infraorbital canal* and gives off the *middle superior alveolar* and *anterior superior alveolar* nerves.

The middle superior alveolar nerve passes downwards in the lateral wall of the maxillary sinus, supplying its mucosa, and forms a plexus with the other superior alveolar nerves. The nerve is present in only 50% of people and, when present, supplies the upper premolar teeth and the mesiobuccal root of the upper first molar. If the nerve is absent these teeth are supplied by the other nerves forming the superior alveolar plexus.

The anterior superior alveolar nerve runs down in the anterior wall of the maxillary sinus, supplying its mucosa, and gives off *posterior* branches which form part of the superior alveolar plexus and supply the upper canine tooth, *nasal* branches which supply the mucosa of a small area of the anterior nasal cavity and *incisive* branches which supply the upper incisor teeth.

The infraorbital nerve emerges onto the face at the *infraorbital foramen* and gives off nasal branches to the skin of the side of the nose, palpebral branches to the skin and conjunctiva of the lower eyelid and a labial branch to the skin and mucous membrane of the upper lip.

3. *Mandibular.* The mandibular division of the trigeminal nerve passes through the foramen ovale as sensory and motor roots to enter the infratemporal fossa where the roots combine to form a single stem. Small branches arise from the stem, a sensory branch, the *nervus spinosus*, re-entering the skull through the foramen spinosum to supply the dura of the middle cranial fossa. The other branches are motor nerves and pass directly to medial pterygoid muscle and indirectly, without synapsing, through the otic ganglion to tensor tympani and tensor palati muscles. The main stem of the nerve divides shortly afterwards into *anterior* and *posterior* divisions.

1. Anterior division

This lies deep to lateral pterygoid muscle and gives off motor branches to masseter, temporalis and lateral pterygoid muscles.

The nerve to masseter passes between the two heads of lateral pterygoid and above the mandibular notch to enter the deep surface of masseter muscle. Temporalis muscle is supplied by two or three branches which emerge above lateral pterygoid and pass upwards deep to temporalis. Two branches, one to each head, supply lateral pterygoid by passing into its deep surface.

The terminal portion of the anterior division emerges between the heads of lateral pterygoid as the *buccal* nerve, passes deep to the coronoid process of the mandible, through the buccal fat pad and onto the surface of buccinator muscle. It is sensory to the mucous membrane and skin of the cheek, and the buccal gum.

2. Posterior division

This lies deep to lateral pterygoid muscle and has three branches as follows.

The *auriculotemporal* nerve passes posteriorly, splits to encircle the middle meningeal artery, lies medial to and then behind the temporomandibular joint, enters a portion of the parotid gland and then passes upwards between the T.M. joint and the external auditory meatus. En route it supplies the capsule and part of the disc of the T.M. joint, the anterior part of the external ear, the external auditory meatus, and the lateral surface of the tympanic membrane.

Postganglionic parasympathetic secretomotor fibres (from the IXth nerve via the tympanic nerve, the tympanic plexus and the lesser superficial petrosal nerve) and *sympathetic* fibres (from the plexus on the middle meningeal artery) pass from the otic ganglion via the auriculotemporal nerve to the parotid gland.

The nerve continues upwards over the root of the zygomatic process and its terminal *temporal* branches supply the skin of the temporal region.

The *lingual* nerve passes downwards and forwards deep to lateral pterygoid, where it is joined by the *chorda tympani* branch of the VIIth nerve, and then superficial to medial pterygoid muscle, entering the floor of the mouth slightly below and posterior to the lower third molar tooth. It passes forwards lateral to hyoglossus muscle, curves under the submandibular duct from the lateral to the medial side, and enters the tongue.

Suspended under the nerve in the region of hyoglossus is the *submandibular ganglion* into which pass *preganglionic parasympathetic* fibres from the VIIth nerve via the chorda tympani and *postganglionic sympathetic* fibres from plexuses associated with the lingual and facial arteries. The parasympathetic fibres synapse here and both types of fibre pass on to supply the submandibular and sublingual salivary glands and the mucous glands of the floor of the mouth and tongue.

The lingual nerve is sensory to the anterior two-thirds of the tongue, the mucous membrane of the floor of the mouth and the lingual gum of the lower teeth. The chorda tympani fibres travelling with it mediate the special sense of taste from the anterior two thirds of the tongue.

The *inferior alveolar* nerve lies deep to lateral pterygoid and runs downwards, behind the lingual nerve, towards the mandibular foramen. Just before it enters the foramen a small branch, the *nerve to mylohyoid*, is given off, which runs downwards to supply motor fibres to mylohyoid muscle and the anterior belly of digastric muscle.

The inferior alveolar nerve enters the mandibular foramen and sends branches to supply sensation to the lower molar and premolar teeth. It divides terminally into the *incisive* nerve, which is the sensory nerve to the lower canine and incisor teeth, and the *mental* nerve, which emerges through the mental foramen to supply sensation to the labial gum above the foramen, and the skin and mucous membrane of the lower lip and chin. There may be a slight overlap in the area supplied by the incisive nerve, supply extending across the midline to the opposite central incisor.

Sensory fibres from the three divisions of the trigeminal nerve pass from their peripheral areas of distribution through the trigeminal ganglion, where their cell bodies are located (except for the cell bodies of proprioceptive fibres), to the sensory root and into the pons. Fibres mediating the sensation of touch end in the main *sensory nucleus* of the Vth nerve which lies laterally in the mid-pons. Fibres subserving pain and temperature sensations pass downwards to form the *spinal tract* of the Vth nerve which extends from the pons into the superficial lateral aspect of the medulla and the upper part of the spinal cord. Fibres forming the spinal tract end in the *spinal nucleus* of the Vth nerve which lies on the medial side of the tract.

Touch fibres, from the main sensory nucleus, and pain and temperature fibres, from the spinal nucleus, cross to the opposite side and pass upwards to the thalamus. Sensory fibres of both types are relayed from there to the sensory cortex.

Some fibres, concerned with reflexes, pass from the spinal nucleus to motor nuclei of the Vth, VIIth and IXth nerves.

Proprioceptive fibres from the T.M. joint, the periodontal ligaments and the muscles of mastication pass along the motor root of the nerve, through the trigeminal ganglion, to their cell bodies which lie in the *mesencephalic nucleus* of the Vth nerve, located near the aqueduct of the midbrain.

Medial to the main sensory nucleus in the pons lies the *motor nucleus* of the Vth nerve which receives upper motor neurone fibres from *both* motor cortices. Its peripheral fibres pass out through the motor root of the nerve.

Clinical considerations

1. Complete division of one trigeminal nerve will result in a unilateral sensory loss over one side of the face and scalp in the area of Vth nerve distribution and paralysis of the muscles of mastication on that side.

Disorders affecting the separate divisions of the nerve and their branches will result in a sensory and/or motor loss in the area supplied by that division or branch.

2. Central (supranuclear) lesions of the motor root on one side do not produce marked effects on the masticatory muscles since the nucleus is *bilaterally* supplied by upper motor neurones, although the *jaw jerk* may be exaggerated following such lesions.

Peripheral lesions of the motor root lead to weakness and atrophy of the muscles of mastication with deviation towards the affected side on opening the jaw, owing to paralysis of the pterygoid muscles on that side.

3. Peripheral nerve damage may be caused by fractures, increasing pressure in the cavernous sinus area by aneurysm and by tumours of the cerebellopontine angle. Central lesions of the brain stem may damage parts of the Vth nerve nuclei and tracts along with damage to other neuroanatomical tract systems. Many syndromes of this type are known but will not be discussed here.

4. *Facial pain* may be a symptom of a number of conditions which involve the trigeminal nerve or the structures it supplies, e.g. multiple sclerosis or neurofibroma of the Vth nerve.

Trigeminal neuralgia is a form of severe, acute, paroxysmal pain of unknown aetiology which is usually confined to the maxillary or mandibular divisions of the nerve. Pain is precipitated by stimulation of a localised 'trigger zone' on the skin or oral mucosa of the affected side by touch, cold air, talking or chewing.

5. A foreign body touching the cornea initiates the *corneal reflex*, with prompt closure of the eyelids. Sensory fibres from the cornea enter the spinal nucleus of the Vth nerve and fibres are relayed from there to both VIIth nerve nuclei whose motor fibres activate the closure of both eyes. Division of the trigeminal nerve causes a loss of both the direct and the consensual corneal reflex. Loss of the direct reflex with preservation of the consensual reflex occurs if the facial nerve on the tested side is destroyed.

Clinical testing of the trigeminal nerve. 1. The various sensory modalities are tested using wisps of cotton wool or paper tissue (touch), pin pricks (pain) and hot and cold objects (temperature) in the areas of distribution of the nerve divisions. Sides are compared.

2. Corneal reflexes are tested by gently touching the cornea with cotton wool. Striking the chin with a tendon hammer when the jaw is open elicits the jaw jerk.

3. Motor function is tested by comparing the contraction and size of masseter and temporalis muscles with the jaw clenched, noting any atrophy or fasciculation present and any deviation of the jaw on opening it against resistance.

Cranial nerve VII (facial)

The facial nerve leaves the brain stem from the lower lateral part of the pons, in the pontocerebellar angle, as a *motor* root and a *sensory* root, the *nervus intermedius*. The *motor* fibres of the facial nerve arise from the *motor nucleus* of the nerve within the lower pons and run in the motor root. *Preganglionic parasympathetic secretomotor* fibres pass from the superior salivatory nucleus of the medulla and run in the sensory root of the nerve. *Sensory* fibres have their cell bodies located in the geniculate ganglion and their central processes pass in the sensory root to the *nucleus of the solitary tract* of the medulla.

The two roots enter the internal auditory meatus, along with the VIIIth nerve, and unite. The VIIth nerve then enters the *facial canal* which passes through the petrous temporal bone, with the semicircular canals lying posteriorly and the cochlea anteriorly, until it reaches the medial wall of the middle ear where it turns sharply backwards and forms the *external genu* or *geniculate ganglion*.

From the genu a branch, the *greater superficial petrosal* nerve, is given off which contains preganglionic parasympathetic and sensory (taste) fibres. It joins the *deep petrosal* nerve, carrying sympathetic fibres, and runs to the sphenopalatine ganglion where the parasympathetic fibres synapse. The postganglionic fibres are distributed from the ganglion to the lacrimal gland via the zygomatic branch of the maxillary nerve, and the mucous membrane of the palate, nasal cavity, and nasopharynx via the nasal, palatal and pharyngeal branches of the maxillary nerve. The taste fibres pass via the greater and lesser palatine nerves to the palate.

The facial nerve then runs backwards across the roof of the middle ear giving off some small *tympanic* branches to the tympanic plexus (along with branches of the IXth nerve). The nerve then descends behind the middle ear giving off a *motor branch* to stapedius muscle of the ear and the *chorda tympani*.

The chorda tympani enters the middle ear and passes forwards, crossing the ear drum close to the handle of the malleus, to exit by the squamotympanic fissure. It joins the lingual nerve deep to lateral pterygoid muscle and contains taste fibres from the anterior two-thirds of the tongue and preganglionic parasympathetic secretomotor fibres which synapse in the submandibular ganglion and pass to the submandibular and sublingual salivary glands and the glands of the tongue and the floor of the mouth.

The VIIth nerve emerges from the skull through the stylomastoid foramen and gives off motor branches to occipitalis muscle, the posterior auricular muscles, the posterior belly of digastric and stylohyoid muscles, before passing into the parotid gland where it divides into *temporofacial* and *cervicofacial* branches.

The five terminal motor branches of the nerve, the *temporal*, *zygomatic*, *buccal*, *mandibular* and *cervical*, are formed within the gland and emerge from its anterior border to radiate across the face and supply buccinator and platysma muscles and the muscles of facial expression.

The motor nucleus of the VIIth nerve receives fibres from *both* motor cortices through the corticobulbar tracts. Crossed fibres pass to the facial muscles which lie below the palpebral fissure, while those above the fissure (mainly frontalis muscle) receive both crossed and uncrossed fibres, i.e. a *bilateral* cortical innervation.

Taste fibres cross and are relayed from the nucleus of the solitary tract via the medial lemniscus and the thalamus to the taste area in the cortex of the postcentral gyrus. Reflex fibres also pass to the salivatory nuclei and the motor nucleus of VII.

Clinical considerations

The effects of damage to the facial nerve vary with the site of the lesion along the course of the nerve.

1. Damage to the nerve where it lies outwith the stylomastoid foramen, for instance in surgical procedures on the parotid gland or in the mastoid area, results in a flaccid paralysis of the muscles of facial expression on that side. At rest this may show up as 'sagging' of the affected side, drooping of the mouth and obliteration of the normal lines of the face. The paralysis is more apparent when an attempt is made to use the affected muscles, with a loss of normal expression on the affected side and deviation of the mouth to the opposite side on smiling.

Paralysis of orbicularis oculi means that the ability to blink the eyelid is lost and this may lead to a drying-out of the eye with possible superinfection and corneal ulceration. Tears may course down the cheek from the eye.

Paralysis of orbicularis oris results in drooling of saliva from the open mouth. Speech and mastication are also affected. Mastication is also affected by paralysis of buccinator muscle, with inability to hold food between the teeth during chewing. Food collects in the affected cheek.

Damage to the individual branches of the nerve, usually by trauma or surgery, will result in paralysis of the area supplied by that branch.

2. Damage to the nerve above its chorda tympani branch results in the signs and symptoms described above plus a loss of taste sensation from the anterior two-thirds of the tongue and a decrease in salivation, both on the affected side.

3. Damage occurring above the nerve branch to stapedius will result in the symptoms and signs described in 1 and 2 above plus *hyperacusis* due to paralysis of stapedius muscle which normally acts to damp down loud and, especially, sudden noises.

4. Involvement of the nerve at the level of the geniculate ganglion will also affect the fibres which travel in the greater superficial petrosal nerve causing a decrease in lacrimation on that side. Pain around the ear is a common symptom at this site of involvement.

5. Damage of the nerve within the internal auditory meatus, e.g. by an acoustic neuroma, may also result in deafness due to involvement of the VIIIth nerve.

6. Upper motor neurone (supranuclear) lesions of the VIIth nerve, usually resulting from cerebral haemorrhage, produce facial paralysis of the muscles below the palpebral fissure, while sparing

those muscles above it. This is due to the fact that these muscles are supplied by fibres from the opposite cerebral cortex also. Paralysis of the lower facial muscles in these lesions is evident in attempts to use them voluntarily but involuntary contractions can still occur, however, since the lower motor neurone remains intact.

Nuclear lesions result in the same type of facial paralysis as the infranuclear lesions described above.

7. Damage to the facial nerve may be due to incorrect deposition of local anaesthetic during inferior alveolar nerve block and is then transient. Involvement by parotid neoplasms or injury during parotid surgery or trauma may occur. Other causes of damage include fractures of the temporal bone, compression in the cerebellopontine angle, acoustic neuroma, infections of the middle ear and herpes zoster of the geniculate ganglion.

Bell's palsy: This condition, of unknown aetiology, is the commonest cause of facial nerve paralysis. It probably arises from inflammation of the nerve within the facial canal and its signs and symptoms are usually that described in 1 above.

Clinical testing of the facial nerve. 1. Observation may reveal asymmetry of the face, flaccidity of the muscles at rest, obliteration of the normal skin folds, deviation of the mouth, drooling and involuntary functioning of the muscles.

2. Motor integrity is tested by asking the patient to smile, frown, shut the eyes tightly, whistle, etc. and comparing the two sides of the face during these actions. Comparison is also made of the muscles above and below the palpebral fissure.

3. Taste sensation may be tested using appropriate substances for the four primary tastes; sugar, salt, quinine and citric acid for the tastes of sweetness, saltiness, bitterness and sourness, respectively.

Cranial nerve VIII (acoustic, vestibulocochlear)

The eighth nerve contains *cochlear* fibres, concerned with hearing, and *vestibular* fibres, concerned with position and balance sense.

Sensory impulses from the organ of Corti, within the cochlea, are relayed along the peripheral fibres of bipolar cells whose cell bodies lie in the *spiral ganglion*, which is located in the central pillar or modiolus of the cochlea. The central processes of these cells form the cochlear component of the VIIIth nerve, which runs through the internal auditory meatus and enters the brainstem between the pons and the medulla.

The cochlear fibres pass to both the *dorsal* and *ventral cochlear* nuclei of the lateral medulla and synapse there. From the dorsal nucleus fibres pass to the opposite lateral lemniscus and from the ventral nucleus fibres pass a) to the opposite lateral lemniscus and b) via the trapezoid bodies and superior olivary nuclei of both sides to *both* lateral lemnisci. The majority of fibres are, therefore, crossed but an uncrossed component is also present.

The lateral lemnisci ascend to the inferior colliculi and then the *medial geniculate bodies*. Fibres pass from the inferior colliculus to nuclei controlling the eye muscles and other cranial and spinal motor nuclei involved in auditory reflexes. Fibres from the medial geniculate body pass to the auditory area of the cortex located on the superior temporal gyrus. The sensory impulses concerned with hearing are represented bilaterally on the temporal cortices.

The peripheral nerve endings of the vestibular fibres of the nerve lie in the ampullae of the semicircular canals and in the maculae of the utricle and saccule. The nerve endings are the peripheral processes of bipolar cells whose cell bodies lie in the *vestibular* ganglion within the internal auditory meatus and whose central processes run with the cochlear fibres to the upper medulla to end in the *vestibular nucleus*, lying in the floor of the fourth ventricle.

Fibres from this nucleus are relayed a) uncrossed to the cerebellum via the inferior cerebellar peduncle, b) uncrossed via the lateral vestibulospinal tract to spinal motor neurones, c) crossed and uncrossed via the medial vestibulospinal tract to cervical spinal motor neurones and d) crossed and uncrossed via the medial longitudinal fasciculi to motor nuclei of the IIIrd, IVth and VIth nerves.

Clinical considerations

1. Damage to the VIIIth nerve by, for example,

skull fracture, tumours, acoustic neuroma, infectious diseases and meningitis, usually results in involvement of both its groups of fibres producing symptoms of both cochlear and vestibular damage.

Bilateral damage to the nerve may be caused by the toxicity of certain drugs, e.g. quinine, aspirin, streptomycin.

2. *Central* lesions involving the auditory pathway on one side do not result in unilateral deafness because of the bilateral representation of hearing on both cortices. The ability to locate the direction from which sounds arise may be lost but no obvious auditory deficit is found.

3. Cochlear fibre damage results in *tinnitus*, a ringing, buzzing or roaring noise in the ear, or, more severely, in *deafness* or impaired hearing on that side. Note that deafness may be due to nerve damage (nerve deafness) but can also be caused by disease of the middle or external ear which interferes with the transmission of sound through the ear (conduction deafness). It is important to distinguish between the two types.

4. Damage to vestibular fibres results in *vertigo*, a feeling of dizziness or whirling in which the patient may falsely feel himself to be moving relative to his surroundings or may feel that his surroundings are moving relative to him, and *nystagmus*, an ocular movement consisting of a slow drift of the eyes towards the affected side followed by a rapid jerk back.

Vertigo may be caused by damage to the vestibular component of the eighth nerve by fractures, acoustic neuroma, drug damage, etc. by conditions affecting the ear, such as otitis media, by cerebellar and brainstem lesions involving the vestibular pathways, Meniere's syndrome (paroxysmal vertigo with tinnitus and deafness, of unknown cause) and seasickness. Nystagmus is due to a disturbance of the vestibulo-ocular pathways but may also occur in cerebellar lesions.

Clinical testing of the vestibulocochlear nerve. 1. Hearing can be crudely tested in each ear, the other being occluded, by the ability to hear whispered words or the ticking of a watch. More accurate measurements of the volume and frequency of sounds heard can be obtained by audiometry.

2. In differentiating between nerve and conduction deafness use is made of the fact that conduc-

tion of sound is normally better through air than through the bone of the skull:

a. *Rinne's test*: A tuning fork is held close to the external auditory meatus until the sound is no longer heard. Its base is then placed onto the mastoid process of that side. If no sound is heard then air conduction is better than bone conduction for that ear and deafness, if present, is of the *nerve deafness* type. If sound is heard then bone conduction is better than air conduction and deafness is of a *conductive* type.

b. *Weber's test*: The base of a tuning fork is held on the vertex of the skull. Normally both ears will hear the sound equally but in conductive deafness sound is referred towards the affected ear and in nerve deafness towards the better ear.

3. The external auditory meatus and the tympanic membrane can be directly visualised using an otoscope. Foreign bodies or wax in the external meatus, perforation of the drum and infections of the middle ear can be seen.

4. Nystagmus may be induced by stimulation of the vestibular system of each ear. Cold water poured into the *right* ear (with the head tilted back at 60° to bring the horizontal semicircular canal into a vertical position) will induce a horizontal nystagmus with its slow component to the *right* and its fast component to the left. Warm water produces the opposite effect. An absent or decreased reaction to this test occurs if vestibular fibres are destroyed.

Cranial nerve IX (glossopharyngeal)

The ninth nerve arises from the upper lateral part of the medulla as three or four rootlets which combine to form a single stem passing to the jugular foramen, by which the nerve exits from the skull. Within the jugular foramen lie the two *sensory ganglia* of the glossopharyngeal nerve.

The nerve passes forwards from the foramen, lying first between the internal jugular vein and the internal carotid artery, and then between the internal and external carotid arteries. It runs forwards on the surface of stylopharyngeus muscle, enters the wall of the pharynx between the superior and middle constrictor muscles, and terminates in the posterior third of the tongue.

Branches of the nerve: The *tympanic* (Jacobson's) nerve is given off within or just below the jugular foramen. It passes in a small bony canal to the middle ear and forms the *tympanic plexus* with part of the VIIth nerve. Sensory branches of the plexus pass to the mucous membrane of the middle ear and auditory tube. *Preganglionic parasympathetic secretomotor* fibres of the IXth nerve pass from the plexus into the *lesser superficial petrosal* nerve.

Sensory *carotid* branches run down on the internal carotid artery to supply the baroreceptors of the carotid sinus and the chemoreceptors of the carotid body.

As the nerve runs along stylopharyngeus muscle a *motor* branch to the muscle is given off.

Within the pharyngeal wall sensory *pharyngeal* branches pass to the *pharyngeal plexus* with branches from the Xth nerve. Sensory branches of the plexus supply the mucous membrane of the pharynx.

Tonsillar branches pass to a plexus around the tonsil and supply sensation to the upper pharynx and the auditory tube.

Finally, *lingual* branches supply general and taste sensation to the mucosa of the posterior third of the tongue.

Motor fibres within the IXth nerve arise from the upper end of the *nucleus ambiguus*, which lies in the lateral medulla, and pass into the branch of the nerve which supplies stylopharyngeus. These fibres are connected to the motor cortex via the corticobulbar tracts.

Parasympathetic fibres have their cell bodies in the *inferior salivatory nucleus* of the medulla. Their preganglionic secretomotor fibres pass via the tympanic nerve, tympanic plexus and lesser superficial petrosal nerve to the *otic ganglion*, where they synapse. Postganglionic fibres pass to the parotid gland via the auriculotemporal nerve. Reflex connections are present between the inferior salivatory nucleus and the nucleus of the solitary tract.

The cell bodies of unipolar glossopharyngeal sensory fibres lie in the sensory ganglia of the nerve. Their peripheral processes for *general* sensation pass to the middle ear, auditory tube, naso- and oropharynx, and the posterior one-third of the tongue via the tympanic, pharyngeal, tonsillar and

lingual nerve branches. The peripheral processes for *chemo-* and *baroreception* pass to the carotid body and sinus, respectively, via the carotid nerve branch; and the peripheral processes for *taste* sensation pass to the posterior one-third of the tongue and the circumvallate papillae via the lingual nerve branch.

The central processes of the general sensory fibres within the IXth nerve enter the medulla and descend to synapse with the *spinal nucleus* of the Vth nerve. Fibres from this nucleus cross and ascend to the thalamus and the sensory cortex; reflex fibres pass to the *nucleus ambiguus*.

Central processes of the glossopharyngeal taste fibres enter the medulla and pass to the upper (gustatory) part of the *solitary tract* and its nucleus. Fibres from this area cross and ascend with the medial lemniscus to the thalamus and then to the cortical taste area. Reflex fibres pass to the inferior salivatory nucleus.

The central processes of the chemo- and baroreceptive fibres pass to the *nucleus* of the solitary tract. Fibres for chemoreception are relayed to the respiratory centre of the medulla, those for baroreception pass to the dorsal motor nucleus of the Xth nerve.

Clinical considerations

1. Taste fibres from both the anterior two-thirds and the posterior one-third of the tongue have reflex connections with the salivatory nuclei and taste impulses can give rise to an increased rate of salivation — the taste: salivation reflex.

2. Increasing blood pressure stimulates the baroreceptors of the carotid sinus and their reflex connections with the Xth nerve produce a decrease in the heart rate. Inhibition of sympathetic cells in the spinal cord produces peripheral vasodilatation and a decrease in blood pressure. In some individuals the sinus is very sensitive to pressure and syncopal attacks may be induced by light pressure on the neck over the sinus.

3. Changes in the concentration of the blood gases stimulate the chemoreceptors of the carotid body. Their central connection with the respiratory centre influences the respiratory rate.

4. Stimulation of the posterior pharyngeal wall excites glossopharyngeal sensory fibres and in-

itiates the *gag reflex*. Reflex connection of these sensory fibres with the nucleus ambiguus stimulates the motor fibres which leave the nucleus via the IXth and Xth nerves to the muscles of the pharynx, larynx and soft palate, causing a contraction and elevation of the palate.

5. Isolated lesions of the glossopharyngeal nerve are rare. Lesions which involve the medulla, e.g. syringobulbia, or the nerve on its course towards or within the jugular foramen, e.g. neoplasm of the posterior cranial fossa, meningitis, thrombophlebitis of the internal jugular vein or trauma, usually involve the Xth and XIth nerves also, due to their proximity to the glossopharyngeal nerve.

Involvement of the IXth nerve will produce a loss of the gag reflex, loss of sensation to the pharynx and the posterior one-third of the tongue, loss of taste sensation to the posterior one-third of the tongue, slight pharyngeal weakness and dysphagia (from paralysis of stylopharyngeus muscle) and possibly loss of salivation from the parotid gland.

Clinical testing of the glossopharyngeal nerve.
1. Sensation of the pharynx and the posterior one-third of the tongue can be tested by touching these areas with a wooden spatula or tongue depressor.

2. The gag reflex can be elicited by touching the posterior wall of the pharynx on either side with the same instrument.

3. Taste sensation to the posterior one-third of the tongue can be tested as for VII.

Cranial nerve X (vagus)

The vagus nerve arises from the lateral part of the medulla, below the IXth nerve, as a number of rootlets. These combine to form the nerve, which passes to the jugular foramen in close relation to the XIth nerve.

Within the foramen the nerve possesses a swelling, the *superior vagal ganglion*, and another swelling is present on the nerve just outside the foramen, the *inferior vagal* (nodose) *ganglion*.

The nerves descend in the neck within the carotid sheaths, lying between the internal jugular veins laterally, and the internal carotid arteries medially. They enter the thoracic cavity, the right nerve passing anterior to the right subclavian artery, and the left nerve passing anterior to the aortic arch between the left common carotid and subclavian arteries. Within the thorax the nerves pass posterior to the hila of the lungs and unite to form the *oesophageal plexus* on the anterior surface of the oesophagus.

From this plexus arise the two vagal trunks, the left lying anterior to the oesophagus, and the right posteriorly, which pass, with the oesophagus, through the diaphragm to enter the abdomen.

Branches of the nerve: Within the jugular foramen the sensory *recurrent meningeal* branch of the nerve arises from the superior ganglion and re-enters the cranial cavity to supply the dura of the posterior cranial fossa.

The *auricular* branch is sensory, passes from the superior ganglion into a canal within the temporal bone, and supplies part of the pinna of the ear, part of the external auditory meatus and the lateral surface of the tympanic membrane.

Three branches arise from the nerve in the region of the inferior ganglion.

The *pharyngeal* branch runs to the pharyngeal plexus (formed by motor fibres from the Xth nerve, sensory fibres from the IXth nerve and sympathetic fibres from the superior cervical ganglion) in the wall of the pharynx. Vagal fibres pass from here to all the pharyngeal and palatal muscles, except stylopharyngeus and tensor palati.

Descending through the neck deep to the internal carotid artery is the *superior laryngeal* nerve. Deep to the superior thyroid artery it divides into an *internal* and an *external laryngeal* branch. The sensory internal laryngeal nerve pierces the thyrohyoid membrane, along with the internal laryngeal artery, and supplies the mucous membrane of the laryngopharynx, the epiglottis and the larynx above the vocal folds. The motor external laryngeal nerve passes downwards to innervate the inferior constrictor and cricothyroid muscles.

The remaining branch from the inferior ganglion is a small sensory *carotid* branch which passes to the wall of the carotid sinus.

Arising from the vagus in the neck is the *cardiac* branch. This runs with the nerve to enter the thorax where it joins the *cardiac plexus*, located below the aortic arch anterior to the bifurcation of the trachea. The cardiac plexus, formed by preganglionic parasympathetic vagal fibres, which synapse within it, and postganglionic sympathetic fibres from the superior and middle cervical ganglia, sends branches to the heart to modify its rate (sympathetic impulses increase heart rate, parasympathetic impulses decrease it).

The *recurrent laryngeal* nerves are branches which arise from the nerves and pass upwards again in the neck.

The right recurrent nerve winds under the right subclavian artery from before backwards, the left recurrent nerve passes similarly under the aortic arch below the ligamentum arteriosum. Both nerves ascend in the neck in the groove between the oesophagus and the trachea and enter the larynx deep to inferior constrictor. They innervate all the intrinsic muscles of the larynx, except cricothyroid, and are sensory to the mucous membrane below the vocal folds.

Behind the hilum of the lung, parasympathetic fibres of the vagus take part in the formation of the *pulmonary plexus* along with sympathetic fibres from the cardiac plexus. Branches of the pulmonary plexus pass to the smooth muscle of the bronchioles (sympathetic impulses dilate the bronchioles, parasympathetic impulses constrict them).

The right and left nerves unite on the anterior surface on the oesophagus to form the *oesophageal plexus*. Postsynaptic parasympathetic vagal fibres pass from the plexus to the smooth muscle and glands of the oesophagus.

The anterior and posterior vagal trunks enter the abdomen and send fibres to the *coeliac, hepatic, splenic* and *renal* plexuses, and from there to abdominal smooth muscle and glands. The anterior trunk, containing fibres mainly from the left vagus nerve, supplies the anterior surface and lesser curvature of the stomach, the liver, gall bladder, duodenum and pancreas. The posterior trunk, mainly right vagal fibres, supplies the posterior surface and greater curvature of the stomach and the midgut and its derivatives up to the left colic flexure.

Motor fibres within the Xth nerve arise from the *nucleus ambiguus* of the medulla. Vagal motor fibres pass via the pharyngeal plexus to the palatal and pharyngeal muscles and via the external laryngeal nerve to the cricothyroid and inferior constrictor muscles.

Also arising from the lower part of the nucleus ambiguus are motor fibres which form the *cranial* root of the XIth nerve. These join the *spinal* root of the XIth nerve and exit through the jugular foramen. Just below the skull, however, the cranial root leaves the spinal root and joins the vagus nerve. Its fibres are distributed via the recurrent laryngeal branches of the vagus to the intrinsic muscles of the larynx.

Vagal *parasympathetic* fibres have their cell bodies in the *dorsal motor nucleus* of the vagus. Their preganglionic fibres pass to the cardiac, pulmonary, oesophageal and abdominal ganglia where they synapse. Their postganglionic fibres pass from these ganglia to the viscera supplied.

Sensory fibres of the Xth nerve are of three types; somatic, visceral and taste fibres.

The cell bodies of vagal *taste* fibres lie in the inferior vagal ganglia. Their peripheral processes pass to the taste buds in the epiglottic region and the laryngeal inlet and their central processes pass to the gustatory part of the solitary tract and its nucleus.

Cell bodies of *visceral* sensory fibres lie in the inferior vagal ganglion. Peripheral processes pass to the pharynx, larynx, trachea, bronchi, oesophagus, heart and abdominal viscera and their central processes to the solitary tract and its nucleus.

The cell bodies of *somatic* sensory fibres lie in the superior vagal ganglion. Their peripheral branches pass to the dura of the posterior fossa via the recurrent meningeal branch, and the external auditory meatus, tympanic membrane and part of the ear via the auricular branch. Central processes of these cells pass to the spinal tract and the nucleus of the spinal tract of the Vth nerve.

Central connections to the nucleus ambiguus are conveyed by the corticobulbar tracts. Reflex fibres pass to it from the solitary tract nucleus.

The dorsal motor nucleus has reflex connections with the solitary tract nucleus and the nucleus of the spinal tract of V.

The nucleus of the solitary tract has reflex connections with the nucleus ambiguus, the salivatory nuclei and the motor nucleus of VII and is connected to the cortex via the medial lemniscus and the thalamus.

The nucleus of the spinal tract of V is connected centrally to the sensory cortex via the thalamus.

Clinical considerations

1. The parasympathetic component of the vagus nerve passes to various plexuses in the thorax and abdomen to innervate the thoracic and most of the abdominal viscera. Stimulation of these fibres will produce a decrease in heart rate, constriction of the bronchioles of the lung, an increase in gut peristalsis, relaxation of the pyloric and ileocaecal sphincters and an increase in secretion from the glands of the bronchi, stomach and pancreas.

2. Sensory impulses from the viscera are carried in the Xth nerve, chiefly the sensation of *nausea*. These sensory fibres are also concerned with the *vomiting reflex*, mediated by connections between the nucleus of the solitary tract and the nucleus ambiguus and the dorsal motor nucleus of the Xth nerve.

Vomiting may also be initiated by pressure on the medulla and the floor of the fourth ventricle either by local factors or a general increase in intracranial pressure.

3. The motor component of the *gag reflex* is mediated by vagal fibres. Paralysis of the vagus leads to a loss of this reflex on the affected side.

4. Irritation of the mucosa of the larynx, trachea or bronchial tree initiates the *cough reflex*. Sensory impulses are relayed to the nucleus of the solitary tract by vagal fibres. Reflex connections pass to the nucleus ambiguus, and thence to the laryngeal and pharyngeal musculature, and to the respiratory centre, to bring about an explosive forced expiration.

5. Isolated lesions of the vagus nerve are uncommon (see IXth nerve) but peripheral involvement of the nerve or its branches in disease of related structures or injury by trauma or at operation may occur.

Paralysis of one vagus nerve usually produces a loss of its somatic functions with little visceral impairment, e.g. paralysis of palatal, pharyngeal and laryngeal muscles on the affected side leading to hoarseness of speech, dysphagia and possibly a degree of dyspnoea. Anaesthesia of the pharynx and larynx will also be present on the same side.

Bilateral involvement of the vagi will result in total laryngeal paralysis, dyspnoea, vomiting, abdominal pain and disturbances to the heart and respiratory rates. Lesions of this sort are fatal.

Damage to the recurrent and superior laryngeal nerves is discussed in the section dealing with the larynx.

6. In the operation of *vagotomy*, the anterior and posterior vagal trunks are divided at the lower end of the oesophagus in an attempt to decrease the level of gastric acid secretion. However, vagatomy also deprives the stomach of its motor supply rendering it atonic. Difficulty in emptying the stomach contents means that vagotomy is usually combined with a stomach-drainage procedure (pyloroplasty or gastrojejunostomy).

Clinical testing of the vagus nerve. 1. The gag reflex is tested as in IX.

2. Sensation of the pharynx and larynx can be tested as in IX.

3. The soft palate can be inspected directly through the open mouth when the patient is asked to say, 'ah'. In unilateral paralysis of the muscles the paralysed side will not elevate and the uvula will be pulled towards the normal side, i.e. *away* from the side of the lesion.

4. Inspection of the larynx and the vocal folds is possible, indirectly, by using a laryngeal mirror. Paralysis of the vocal folds can be seen during attempts at phonation.

Cranial nerve XI (accessory)

The accessory nerve arises from two roots. The *cranial* root arises from the medulla as four or five filaments below the origin of the vagus nerve. It is joined, within the skull, by the *spinal* root, which arises as fibres from the spinal segments C1–5, which join to form a trunk which ascends through the foramen magnum. The XIth nerve leaves the skull through the jugular foramen with the IXth and Xth nerves.

The cranial root leaves the accessory nerve to join the vagus nerve at the inferior vagal ganglion and its fibres are distributed to the intrinsic muscles of the larynx (except cricothyroid muscle) via the recurrent laryngeal branches of the vagus.

The spinal root passes backwards over the internal jugular vein to enter the sternomastoid muscle, which it supplies, before passing downwards and backwards across the posterior triangle of the neck to enter the deep surface of trapezius muscle, which it also supplies.

The fibres of the cranial root of the nerve arise from the lower part of the *nucleus ambiguus* of the medulla, those of the spinal root have their cell bodies located in the anterior horns of the first five cervical segments of the spinal cord. The nucleus ambiguus is connected to the motor cortex via the corticobulbar tracts and receives reflex fibres from the nucleus of the solitary tract. The cervical fibres are lower motor neurones and have similar connections with the cortex via the corticospinal tracts as any other cells of this type.

Clinical considerations

1. Isolated lesions of the cranial root are rare and this portion of the nerve may be involved in lesions which affect the IXth and Xth nerves also. Damage to the vagus nerve, particularly its recurrent laryngeal branches (see vagus), may affect fibres of the cranial root of the XIth nerve.

2. Lesions involving the spinal root of the nerve, e.g. trauma to, or operation upon, the posterior triangle, result in paralysis and atrophy of sternomastoid and trapezius muscles with an inability to turn the head *away* from the affected side and to shrug the shoulder on the affected side.

3. In upper motor neurone lesions, spasticity of the muscles but no atrophy is present and, in unilateral damage, a *torticollis* (wry neck), may result.

4. Torticollis may be congenital, following fibrosis within one sternomastoid muscle after haematoma, or may be due to local disease or trauma. *Spasmodic* torticollis, with involuntary neck movements, may be caused by extrapyramidal disease, and may be unresponsive to any treatment other than surgical division of the spinal accessory nerve.

Clinical testing of the accessory nerve. 1. For tests of the cranial root, see X.

2. To test the integrity of the spinal root the patient is examined for atrophy or wasting of sternomastoid and trapezius muscles and drooping of the shoulder. The power of trapezius is tested by asking the patient to shrug his shoulders against resistance, and comparing sides. Pressing the chin down against resistance outlines the sternomastoid

muscles. Deviation may be noticed *toward* the affected side during this procedure. The individual sternomastoid muscles are tested by rotating the head against resistance to either side. Paralysis or weakness is noticed on an attempt to turn the head *away* from the affected side.

Cranial nerve XII (hypoglossal)

The hypoglossal nerve arises from between the pyramid and olive of the medulla as a number of filaments which combine and pass laterally to traverse the *hypoglossal canal* and enter the neck.

In the neck the nerve lies within the carotid sheath and passes downwards between the internal jugular vein and the internal carotid artery. At about the level of the angle of the mandible it passes forwards superficial to the external carotid artery and its lingual and facial branches, and enters the mouth between the hyoglossus muscle medially and mylohyoid muscle laterally. Anterior to hyoglossus it runs medially to enter the tongue.

The XIIth nerve supplies all the intrinsic and extrinsic muscles of the tongue, except palatoglossus.

The nerve is joined at the base of the skull by fibres from the anterior ramus of C1. These fibres run with the XIIth nerve and give off the following branches.

A recurrent *meningeal* branch passes upwards through the hypoglossal canal to supply sensation to the dura of the posterior cranial fossa.

Motor *muscular* branches pass to geniohyoid and thyrohyoid muscles.

The *descendens hypoglossi* passes downwards along the carotid sheath to form a loop, at the level of the larynx, with fibres from the anterior rami of C2 and C3, which descend as the *descendens cervicalis*. The loop is termed the *ansa hypoglossi*, and motor branches from it pass to the sternohyoid, sternothyroid and omohyoid muscles.

The motor fibres of the hypoglossal nerve arise from the *hypoglossal nucleus*, situated near the midline of the medulla in the floor of the IVth ventricle. The nucleus receives crossed cortical fibres via the corticobulbar tracts and reflex fibres from the trigeminal sensory nuclei and the nucleus of the solitary tract.

Clinical considerations

1. The XIIth nerve may be damaged by trauma at or below its exit from the skull, e.g. skull fracture, upper cervical fracture or dislocation. The hypoglossal nucleus or its central connections may be involved in intracranial lesions, e.g. haemorrhage, tumour, syringobulbia, multiple sclerosis, infections of the posterior cranial fossa, etc.

2. Peripheral damage to the nerve, or damage to its nucleus, causes a flaccid paralysis of the muscles of the tongue on the affected side, atrophy of the paralysed muscles with 'wrinkling' of the tongue on that side, and deviation of the tongue *towards* the side of the lesion on protrusion. Fasciculation of the affected half of the tongue may also be present.

Involvement of the hypoglossal nucleus is usually associated with damage to related nerves or medullary structures.

3. Supranuclear damage, e.g. lesions of the corticobulbar tracts, results in a spastic paralysis, without wasting or fibrillation, to the contralateral side of the tongue.

4. Hemiparalysis of the tongue may give rise to difficulty with speech, mastication and swallowing.

Clinical testing of the hypoglossal nerve. 1. Observation of the tongue may reveal wasting, wrinkling or fasciculation. Deviation of the tongue on protrusion should be noted.

2. The power of the tongue musculature can be tested by asking the patient to push each cheek out with his tongue against resistance. Comparison of both sides can be made.

THE AUTONOMIC NERVOUS SYSTEM

The autonomic nervous system is part of the peripheral nervous system and is essentially an involuntary or automatic motor system, requiring no conscious control. It innervates smooth muscle, notably in the vascular and digestive systems, and controls the secretion of many glands.

It consists of *sympathetic* and *parasympathetic* divisions both characterised by being formed of a two-neuron chain. The primary or *preganglionic* neuron has its cell body located within the central nervous system, it synapses with the cell body of the secondary or *postganglionic* neuron in an autonomic *ganglion* outwith the central nervous system and the fibres of the secondary neuron pass from there to the effector organ. Many organs receive fibres from both components of the autonomic nervous system and are said to possess a *dual innervation*.

Sympathetic division

The cell bodies of sympathetic preganglionic neurons lie in the lateral horns of grey matter present in the thoracic and the upper two lumbar segments of the spinal cord (T1 to L2). The fibres of these cells leave the cord through the anterior roots and join the spinal nerves of these segments. The sympathetic nervous system is said, therefore, to have a *thoracolumbar* outflow.

The ganglia of the sympathetic nervous system form two groups. One group, the *paravertebral* ganglia, lie alongside the vertebral column throughout its length. They are joined together by nerve fibres and form the sympathetic *trunk* or *chain*. The other group of ganglia lie anterior to the vertebral column in the abdomen, close to the large abdominal arteries after which they are named (coeliac, superior and inferior mesenteric ganglia). These are *prevertebral* ganglia.

Both groups receive sympathetic preganglionic fibres which leave the spinal nerves T1 to L2 via *white rami communicantes* which join the spinal nerves to a ganglion of the sympathetic chain. The white rami are so named because they contain myelinated fibres. Fibres within a white ramus may a) synapse within the sympathetic ganglion to which they pass, b) pass up or down the chain for variable distances before synapsing within a ganglion or c) pass through the ganglion without synapsing to form *splanchnic nerves* which pass to the prevertebral ganglia and then synapse.

Postganglionic sympathetic fibres reach their destinations in one of three ways, as follows.

Postganglionic fibres from the prevertebral ganglia pass to the abdominal viscera via autonomic *plexuses* associated with branches of the abdominal aorta. The thoracic splanchnic nerves, containing preganglionic fibres, synapse in the coeliac and superior mesenteric ganglia and supply fore- and midgut derivatives via the coeliac plexus; the lumbar splanchnic nerves, also containing pre-ganglionic fibres, synapse in the inferior mesenteric ganglion and supply structures derived from the hindgut and the urogenital tract via the hypogastric plexus.

Postganglionic fibres from the paravertebral ganglia of the sympathetic chain may pass via the cardiac and pulmonary plexuses to the thoracic organs or from the superior cervical ganglion via the internal and external carotid plexuses to the head and neck.

Most of the postganglionic fibres, however, pass from the ganglia of the chain to all the spinal nerves via the *grey rami communicantes* (containing unmyelinated fibres) and go on to supply the sweat glands and smooth muscle in blood vessels and around hair follicles all over the body. It follows that there are more grey rami than white since the sympathetic chain is connected to each spinal nerve by a grey ramus whereas only the spinal nerves T1 to L2 possess white rami.

Sympathetic supply to the head

The sympathetic chain in the neck lies deep to the prevertebral fascia on the prevertebral muscles. Anterior to it lies the carotid sheath and its contents.

The cervical chain is made up of sympathetic fibres which have arisen as white rami from thoracic spinal nerves and ascended to synapse within the cervical ganglia. There are three of these ganglia in the cervical region.

1. The *inferior cervical* ganglion lies near the subclavian artery and gives off postganglionic fibres which are distributed with the subclavian and vertebral arteries, as grey rami communicantes which join the spinal nerves C7 and C8, and fibres which pass downwards to the cardiac plexus.

2. The *middle cervical* ganglion lies at the level of the cricoid cartilage and its postganglionic fibres are distributed to the thyroid gland along the inferior thyroid artery, as grey rami communicantes which join the spinal nerves C5 and C6, and fibres which join the cardiac plexus.

3. The *superior cervical* ganglion is large and lies near the base of the skull giving off postganglionic fibres as grey rami communicantes which join the spinal nerves C1 to C4, fibres which pass to the cardiac plexus, fibres which pass to the thyroid gland, and fibres which form the carotid plexuses around the internal and external carotid arteries and are distributed with their branches.

Sympathetic fibres run with branches of the external carotid artery to the skin and tissues of the face, the scalp, the salivary glands and the mucous membrane of the nasal and oral cavities. Sympathetic fibres are distributed with the internal carotid artery to the orbit, lacrimal gland and the cranial cavity.

Sympathetic fibres also pass to the pharyngeal plexus, to cranial nerves IX, X, XI and XII and to the cranial parasympathetic ganglia — the ciliary, sphenopalatine, otic and submandibular ganglia. No synapses of sympathetic nerves occur within these ganglia.

Parasympathetic division

The cell bodies of preganglionic parasympathetic neurons lie in brainstem nuclei and in the grey matter of the sacral spinal cord segments S2 to S4. The parasympathetic nervous system is therefore said to have a *craniosacral* outflow.

The sacral preganglionic parasympathetic fibres pass as the *pelvic splanchnic* nerves to the hypogastric plexus, where some of the ganglia lie, and are distributed to the terminal part of the digestive tract and to the genitourinary tract. Most of the parasympathetic ganglia lie close to or within the organs supplied and are termed *terminal* or *intramural* ganglia. Their postganglionic fibres are therefore very short, for the most part.

The cranial preganglionic parasympathetic fibres run with the IIIrd, VIIth, IXth and Xth cranial nerves.

Vagal preganglionic parasympathetic fibres are distributed to the heart and lungs via the cardiac and pulmonary plexuses, to the oesophagus via the oesophageal plexus and to the abdominal viscera and derivatives of the fore- and midgut via the coeliac plexus, which contains some of the ganglia, and the right and left vagal trunks.

Parasympathetic supply to the head

Preganglionic parasympathetic fibres of the oculomotor, facial and glossopharyngeal nerves pass to four pairs of cranial parasympathetic ganglia in the head, lying close to the organs that they innervate. These are the ciliary, sphenopalatine, otic and submandibular ganglia and within them the preganglionic parasympathetic fibres synapse with the cell bodies of postganglionic parasympathetic fibres. Each ganglion also receives postganglionic sympathetic fibres and sensory fibres from one of the divisions of the trigeminal nerve. These pass through the ganglion without synapsing.

Ciliary ganglion

Located in the orbit on the lateral side of the optic nerve, this ganglion receives parasympathetic fibres from the IIIrd nerve, sympathetic fibres from the plexus around the internal carotid and ophthalmic arteries and sensory fibres from the nasociliary nerve. The fibres are distributed via the *short ciliary* nerves to the eyeball.

The postganglionic parasympathetic fibres pass to the ciliary and sphincter pupillae muscles, the sympathetic fibres to the ocular vessels and dilator pupillae muscle and the sensory fibres to the eyeball.

Sphenopalatine ganglion

This ganglion hangs down from the maxillary nerve in the pterygopalatine fossa. It receives preganglionic parasympathetic fibres from the VIIth nerve which travel from the geniculate ganglion via the greater superficial petrosal and Vidian nerves, sympathetic fibres from the internal carotid plexus via the deep petrosal and Vidian nerves and sensory fibres from the maxillary nerve, facial nerve and glossopharyngeal nerve (via the tympanic plexus).

The postganglionic parasympathetic fibres pass to the lacrimal gland via the zygomatic branch of the maxillary nerve and the lacrimal branch of the ophthalmic division of the trigeminal nerve, and to the glands of the nasal cavity, pharyngeal roof and palate via the nasal, pharyngeal and palatine branches of the maxillary nerve. Sympathetic and sensory fibres pass to the mucosa of the nasal cavity, palate and roof of the pharynx.

Otic ganglion

This ganglion lies on the medial side of the mandibular nerve just below the foramen ovale. It receives pre-ganglionic parasympathetic fibres from the IXth nerve via the tympanic nerve, tympanic plexus and the lesser superficial petrosal nerve. Sympathetic fibres enter the ganglion from the plexus on the middle meningeal artery and sensory fibres pass to the ganglion from the mandibular nerve and from the VIIth and IXth nerves via the tympanic plexus and the lesser superficial petrosal nerve.

Sympathetic, sensory and postganglionic parasympathetic fibres travel from the ganglion to the parotid gland via the auriculotemporal nerve.

Trigeminal motor fibres from the mandibular nerve also traverse the otic ganglion, without synapsing, to supply tensor tympani and tensor palati muscles.

Submandibular ganglion

Hanging from the lingual nerve in the floor of the mouth lies the submandibular ganglion which receives preganglionic parasympathetic fibres from the VIIth nerve via the chorda tympani and the lingual nerve, sympathetic fibres from the plexus around the facial and lingual arteries and sensory fibres from the lingual nerve and chorda tympani.

Postganglionic parasympathetic fibres pass to the submandibular and sublingual salivary glands. Sensory and sympathetic fibres pass to these salivary glands as well as to the glands and vessels of the oral cavity.

Autonomic afferents

The autonomic nervous system is, by definition, a motor system, but both parasympathetic and sympathetic divisions seem to possess *sensory* components also. The sensory fibres of the sympathetic and sacral parasympathetic components have their cell bodies in the dorsal root ganglia and they travel to the cord in one of two ways.

1. Sympathetic fibres from the periphery travel within the spinal nerves to the spinal cord.

2. Sympathetic and parasympathetic fibres from the viscera travel back within the splanchnic

nerves, ganglia and plexuses which convey autonomic *motor* fibres from the c.n.s.

Cranial parasympathetic sensory fibres have their cell bodies within the sensory ganglia of the parasympathetic cranial nerves and their fibres pass back within these nerves to their nuclei.

Clinical considerations

1. The sympathetic nervous system is mainly concerned with activities that expend energy, especially apparent during stress. It produces dilatation of the pupil, vasoconstriction of the skin and viscera with blood being diverted to the musculature, an increased pulse and blood pressure and constriction of the sphincters. It can be termed a 'fight or flight' system since it prepares the body for either of these situations.

The parasympathetic nervous system, on the other hand, usually produces the opposite effects, being concerned with activities that restore and conserve body energy. It can be termed a 'rest or repose' system since it is active when the body is not outwardly so.

2. *Horner's syndrome.* Involvement of the fibres of the cervical sympathetic chain in the upper thoracic spinal cord by, e.g. pressure from a tumour or syringo-myelia or damage to the cervical part of the sympathetic chain itself by trauma, at operation, by invasion or pressure of a tumour in the neck or upper mediastinum or by pressure from a carotid aneurysm may give rise to a condition known as Horner's syndrome. This gives rise to unilateral pupillary constriction, ptosis and enophthalmos and a dry, flushed face on the affected side and is due to a loss of sympathetic innervation to the affected side of the head.

3. Division of the sympathetic fibres to an area results in a loss of vasoconstrictor and sudomotor functions within that area and leads, as in Horner's syndrome, to a dry, hot, flushed skin in that area. States of excessive sweating (hyperhidrosis), especially of the palms of the hands and the soles of the feet, can therefore be relieved by severing the sympathetic supply to the upper or lower limbs in the operations of cervical or lumbar sympathectomy.

Nerves related to the cavernous venous sinus

A number of nerves pass through the cavernous sinuses, which lie on either side of the body of the sphenoid bone. The oculomotor and trochlear nerves, and the ophthalmic division of the trigeminal nerve, enter the posterior aspect of the sinus and pass forwards in its lateral wall to leave the sinus anteriorly and pass through the superior orbital fissure into the orbit.

The maxillary division of the trigeminal nerve enters the posterior aspect of the sinus, runs in the lower part of the lateral wall and then passes out of the lower part of the sinus to enter the foramen rotundum.

The abducens nerve enters the posterior aspect of the sinus, passes through the sinus with the internal carotid artery medial to it for most of its passage, and exits through the superior orbital fissure. Sympathetic fibres from the cervical ganglia pass with the internal carotid artery and its branches.

Clinical considerations

The close relationship of these nervous structures to the cavernous sinus, and to each other, makes them liable to damage in the following ways.

1. Infections of the superficial or deep tissues of the face, of the orbit or nasal sinuses may spread via the ophthalmic veins or pterygoid venous plexus to involve the cavernous sinus. Such infection may proceed to cavernous sinus thrombophlebitis with subsequent blockage of the venous drainage from the orbit. Clinically, this presents as pain behind the eye, exophthalmos, oedema of the eyelids and conjunctiva, papilloedema and engorgement of the ocular vessels and ocular palsies from involvement of the nerves related to the sinus.

The infection may spread via the intercavernous sinuses to the cavernous sinus of the opposite side. Treatment is by appropriate antibiotic and anticoagulant therapy.

2. The nerves in this area lie close together, especially at the superior orbital fissure, and may be damaged by trauma at this site or by compression from a local tumour. Expanding pituitary tumours

may involve the nerves in the cavernous sinus also, particularly the abducens nerve which lies nearest the pituitary fossa.

3. The abducens nerve is also liable, as are the other nerves related to the sinus, to damage in disorders affecting the internal carotid artery, e.g. aneurysm or arteriovenous fistula between the artery and the cavernous sinus.

PAIN

Physiology

Pain is one of the cutaneous senses and it arises by stimulation of the pain receptors or nociceptors located almost everywhere in the body. The receptors for pain sensation consist of naked nerve endings.

An appropriate stimulus to a receptor produces an increase in the permeability of the cell membrane to Na^+, resulting in an influx of Na^+ into the cell, depolarisation, and the production of an *action potential*. The membrane then repolarises, ready to fire again if the stimulus is repeated. A constantly maintained stimulus results in repeated firings but leads to *adaptation*, where the frequency of production of action potentials decreases over a period of time. Adaptation in pain receptors is, however, very slow.

The sensation of pain is transmitted to the c.n.s. by two types of nerve fibres. One type, A δ fibres, are myelinated fibres of small diameter (2–5 μm), which conduct at 12–30 m/s; the other type, dorsal root C fibres, are unmyelinated, smaller (0.4–1.2 μm), and conduct impulses at a slower rate (0.5–2 m/s).

The larger A δ fibres appear to be concerned with sharp and localised pain, so-called 'fast' pain; the smaller C fibres with more diffuse, aching, 'slow' pain. Type C fibres are less susceptible to blockage by hypoxia and pressure but more susceptible to blockage by local anaesthetic agents.

Pain pathways

Pain fibres, except for those of the head which lie within the cranial nerves, enter the spinal cord via the posterior roots of the spinal nerves. Their cell bodies lie within the dorsal root ganglia and their central processes synapse with cells in the dorsal horns of grey matter. The fibres of these dorsal horn cells soon cross the midline in the anterior white commissure and ascend in the *lateral spinothalamic tract* to a) the ventroposterolateral nucleus of the thalamus and thence to the sensory cortex of the postcentral gyrus and b) the reticular formation and intralaminar nuclei of the thalamus.

The majority of pain fibres from the head lie in the divisions of the trigeminal nerve which provide much of the sensory supply to the skin of the face and scalp. However, the glossopharyngeal nerve, supplying the naso- and oropharynx, the posterior one-third of the tongue, the middle ear and the inner surface of the eardrum and the pharyngotympanic tube, the vagus nerve, supplying part of the external ear and outer surface of the eardrum, the laryngopharynx and larynx, the great auricular nerve, supplying an area of skin over the angle of the mandible and part of the external ear and other branches of the cervical plexus supplying the skin of the neck and scalp also contribute. Where the areas of distribution of these nerves abut onto each other some overlap may occur.

Pain fibres of the trigeminal nerve enter the pons and pass downwards to form the *spinal tract* of the Vth nerve. They terminate in the *spinal nucleus* of the nerve. Fibres from this nucleus cross the brain stem and ascend as the *anterior trigeminothalamic tract* to the ventroposteromedial nucleus of the thalamus and from there to the postcentral gyrus. The trigeminal pathways are also linked to the motor nuclei of the IIIrd, Vth, VIIth, IXth, Xth and XIth cranial nerves and activate various muscular reflexes in response to pain, to the cardiac and respiratory centres, initiating hyperventilation and tachycardia, to the hypothalamopituitary axis, activating the endocrine system, and the reticular formation and limbic system which seem to play a role in the emotional response to pain.

The perception of pain occurs at the level of the thalamus and destruction of the sensory cortex does not eliminate pain.

The trigeminothalamic tract is closely related to the lateral spinothalamic tract in the pons and midbrain and lesions in this area may affect both tracts.

Fibres in the lateral spinothalamic tract are arranged in a logical sequence with those from the cervical segments lying medially and those from lower segments lying more and more laterally. Pressure from outwith the cord by, for example, tumour, will therefore tend to compress the fibres from the lower segments, resulting in a loss of pain sensation from these areas, whereas pressure from tumours within the cord will tend to affect the fibres from the higher segments first.

Visceral pain

The pain receptors of the autonomic nervous system are located within the viscera and pass to the c.n.s. via the sympathetic and parasympathetic divisions. Visceral afferent fibres entering the spinal cord travel in the spinothalamic tracts, those of the head travel with the VIIth, IXth and Xth nerves.

Visceral pain is diffuse and poorly localised since there are few receptors. The receptors are particularly sensitive to distension and the pain produced can be severe. It is associated with nausea and vomiting. Radiation of the pain, referred pain, to other areas also occurs.

Referred pain

Deep somatic pain and visceral pain are both frequently referred. Visceral pain is usually referred to a somatic area which shares the same embryonic site of development, for example, the diaphragm which develops in the neck before migrating caudally is supplied by the phrenic nerve arising from the spinal roots C2, 3 and 4. Irritation of the diaphragm may result in pain being referred to the tip of the shoulder in dermatomes which share the same spinal roots.

The mechanism by which this referral takes place may be explained by the fact that visceral and somatic fibres entering the same spinal root both pass to the spinothalamic tract and, since there are more peripheral sensory fibres than axons within the tract, visceral and somatic fibres may converge upon the same neuron misleading the brain into thinking that the pain arises not from a viscus, but from a somatic area.

Pain can also be referred by nerves which are shared by different tissues, for example, maxillary sinusitis may irritate the superior alveolar nerves, which supply this area of mucosa, and result in pain being referred to nearby teeth since the nerve supply to both areas is the same.

Other examples of pain referral include: cardiac pain (angina) may be referred to the neck and jaw, pain originating in the arteries of the face or in the intracranial venous sinuses may be referred to areas of the face and head, pain from the T.M. joint or the muscles of mastication may be referred to the face and, conversely, pain originating in the stylomastoid muscle may be referred to the T.M. joint area.

Craniofacial pain

Pain felt in the head and neck is a common symptom and in most cases such pain is due to an easily diagnosed and detectable condition such as dental caries or an impacted molar tooth. However, the causes of craniofacial pain are legion and in some cases difficult to diagnose since the pain may be diffuse or poorly localised, atypical in its nature or be referred from another, possibly distant, site. A few causes of craniofacial pain are briefly touched upon below.

Teeth and associated tissues

The pain receptors of the teeth are located within the dental pulp. They may be stimulated by pressure, heat or cold, or by inflammation which is usually the result of dental caries. Stimulation of the pulpal pain receptors, by whichever cause, results in a sharp sensation of pain.

Apical abscesses stimulate both the pulpal pain receptors and the pain and pressure receptors of the periodontal ligament. Pain of this type tends to be dull and throbbing and is increased by pressure or tapping on the affected tooth. The pain may diminish should the abscess rupture since the pressure within it then falls.

Inflammation of the gum, gingivitis, stimulates gum pain receptors. Pain may also be caused by unerupted or impacted teeth.

Abnormal occlusion, bruxism and stress resulting in habits such as teeth clenching, grinding and tapping may lead to pain either within the teeth or in the T.M. joint or masticatory musculature.

Oral cavity and associated tissues

Stomatitis, trauma, burns or infection of the oral mucosa may all produce pain.

Aphthous ulcers, carcinoma and vitamin deficiency states may produce a painful tongue.

The ducts of the salivary glands may become blocked by calculus resulting in pain from the dilated duct proximal to the obstruction. Such pain is more pronounced before meals. Infections of the glands, either superimposed upon obstruction or viral in origin (mumps), tumours of the glands, the oropharynx or the floor of the mouth may also cause pain.

Nasal cavity and paranasal sinuses

An invasive tumour in the lateral wall of the nasopharynx may spread laterally between the skull base and the uppermost fibres of superior constrictor muscle, giving rise to a collection of signs and symptoms known as *Trotter's syndrome*, with pain in the mandible and tongue, decreased palatal movement and deviation of the palate to the affected side.

Of the paranasal sinuses, the maxillary sinuses are most commonly involved in disease processes. Pain may be caused by sinusitis, involvement of the sinus in disease of dental origin or by neoplasm. Pain may be felt in the sinus itself and elicited by pressure over the maxilla on the affected side or may be referred to the upper teeth. Conversely, disease of these teeth may present as a painful maxillary sinus.

Disease of the ethmoid sinuses caused by infection, tumour or congenital abnormalities such as a dermoid cyst may cause pain which is located behind the eye or at the root of the nose. The orbit itself may become involved by a spreading ethmoidal infection or neoplasm.

Disease of the frontal and sphenoidal sinuses may cause pain in the forehead or a basal headache, respectively, although many unusual and bizzarre symptoms may be produced by involvement of the sphenoid sinus due to its close proximity to many important nervous and vascular intracranial structures.

T.M. joint and the muscles of mastication

Pain in the T.M. joint may arise from disease of the joint structures themselves, from the associated musculature or by referral from more distant sites. It is typically dull, diffuse and poorly localised and may radiate to other areas, e.g. temporal area, jaws and teeth. The diagnosis of pain in this area may be difficult.

Involvement of the joint structures, the capsule, synovium and the disc may be due to trauma, degeneration or inflammation. Inflammatory states include infections and rheumatoid arthritis of the joint. Degenerative states include osteoarthritis. Trauma to the joint may arise in a number of ways; by direct blows to the jaw; by excessive opening of the jaw with stretching of the capsule and ligaments during intubation for general anaesthesia or during extraction of lower third molars under general anaesthesia or as a result of a whiplash injury; malocclusion of the teeth may result in joint trauma as may tooth extraction followed by overclosure. Pain in the latter case arises from pressure on the receptors which are located mainly in the posterior part of the articular disc.

Pain may also arise from trauma of the muscles of mastication, either directly or as a result of overstretching of the muscles by excessive contraction in states of stress.

Orbit and ear

In disease processes involving the ear, e.g. otitis media or tumour, pain may be felt locally or can be referred to other areas which share the same nerve supply, i.e. the Vth, IXth and Xth cranial nerves. Referred pain from the various compartments of the ear may therefore be felt in the face, pharynx and larynx. Conversely, pain arising from these sites may be referred to the ear.

Similarly, diseases of the eyeball and the orbit may cause referred pain over the distribution of the ophthalmic division of the trigeminal nerve.

Headache

A large variety of disorders may give rise to headache. Amongst them are conditions affecting the eye and orbit, the ear, the nose and paranasal sinuses, the teeth and related structures, maxillofacial trauma, invasive tumours of the maxillary sinus and nasopharynx, intracranial infection of facial, dental or sinus origin, bruxism, and trigeminal and glossopharyngeal neuralgias.

Headache, especially of the migrainous or 'cluster' type, may cause pain which is referred to the maxilla, behind the eye or to the temporal area.

Nervous structures

Craniofacial pain in the categories mentioned above arises as a result of stimulation of nerve endings. Pain may also be caused by trauma to the nerves or by disease involving the nerves (primary and secondary neuralgias).

Causalgia is a severe, burning pain, which may be associated with trophic changes in the skin, and which follows incomplete tearing of the affected nerve. It may occur after mandibular or facial fractures, in which the inferior alveolar and infraorbital nerves are involved, respectively, or following extraction of the teeth.

Phantom pain, similar to that felt after limb amputation, may occur after tooth extraction also.

Pain, among other symptoms, may occur after division of the facial or auriculotemporal nerves in parotidectomy or in injuries to the parotid area of the face.

Primary neuralgias are diseases of unknown cause, which, in the face, affect the trigeminal and, more rarely, the glossopharyngeal nerves. *Trigeminal neuralgia* is a form of unilateral, severe, acute and paroxysmal pain of unknown cause. It is usually confined to the area of distribution of one of the divisions of the Vth nerve, the maxillary and mandibular divisions being most commonly affected although two or all three of the divisions may be involved together. It occurs in later life, affecting twice as many women as men. The pain felt is initially of short duration but may be present for longer and longer periods of time as the disease progresses. Pain is often precipitated by stimulation of a localised 'trigger zone' on the skin or oral mucosa of the affected side by touch, cold air, talking or chewing. Treatment is with the anticonvulsant drug, carbamazepine or, if this fails, by surgical procedures such as phenol or alcohol injection into the trigeminal ganglion or preganglionic section of the sensory root of the nerve.

Glossopharyngeal neuralgia is similar to trigeminal neuralgia in its symptoms, although the pain is felt in the area of distribution of the IXth nerve, i.e. the tonsillar area, the posterior part of the tongue, the soft palate or the ear. The 'trigger zone' usually lies in the lateral pharyngeal wall, the base of the tongue or the external ear. Pharmacologically the treatment is as for trigeminal neuralgia, surgically the nerve may be sectioned either in the neck or intracranially.

Secondary neuralgias occur when a nerve or its central tracts are involved by an encroaching pathological process. Examples include infiltration of or pressure upon a nervous structure by a spreading neoplasm of nearby tissues or by compression of the nerve or its branches at their exiting foramina by Paget's disease of bone. The pain of secondary neuralgias may mimic that caused by a primary neuralgia of the same nerve making a diagnosis difficult.

Herpetic neuralgia: herpes zoster is a viral infection of dorsal root ganglia causing pain and an erythematous, vesicular rash over the cutaneous distribution of the affected root. Pain may occur before, during or after the attack. Damage to the involved nerve tissue may give rise to a long-lasting neuralgia, *postherpetic neuralgia*, or anaesthesia or parasthesia of the affected nerve or segment. Herpes zoster commonly affects the dorsal root ganglia of the nerves of the trunk with a subsequent and characteristic 'girdle' distribution of vesicles. Infections involving the trigeminal and geniculate ganglia may also occur.

In trigeminal herpes the ophthalmic division is commonly affected, with pain along its area of distribution. Corneal vesicles may appear leading to ulceration of the cornea and possible scarring with visual impairment.

In herpes of the geniculate ganglion of the facial nerve, pain is felt in or behind the ear and may radiate to the face and neck. Vesicles occur on the external ear and intraorally on the mucosa of the oropharynx, the *Ramsey-Hunt syndrome*. Swelling of the ganglion may lead to a Bell's palsy. Spread of the infection may also occur to involve the VIIIth nerve, leading to deafness or vertigo.

Other conditions of nervous structures which may give rise to facial pain include Bell's palsy (see VIIth cranial nerve) and psychiatric disturbances in which atypical facial pain with an unanatomical distribution and no obvious cause may be a symptom.

5

Soft tissues of the face

GENERAL CONSIDERATIONS

The bones of the facial skeleton are covered by extremely mobile soft tissues. In various regions, the forehead, the orbital margins, the bridge of the nose and the zygomatic bone, the covering layer of soft tissue is relatively thin and the underlying bone may be easily palpated. The remarkable mobility of these soft tissues is due to the absence of an inextensible layer of *deep fascia*, except for an area bounded by the angle of the mandible, the zygoma and the external auditory meatus, where the parotid gland is overlain by the parotid fascia, which is an upward extension of the investing layer of the deep cervical fascia.

Subcutaneous fat in the soft tissues softens the contours of the face; over the lateral surface of buccinator muscle subcutaneous fat is present as a thick pad — the *buccal pad of fat*. This is well developed in infants and accounts for the cherubic appearance of the newborn. Elsewhere, the amount of subcutaneous fat varies and, together with underlying differences in the shape of the facial skeleton, accounts for the variation in individual facial appearance.

The face is richly endowed with sensory nerves from the Vth cranial (trigeminal) nerve especially around the facial openings, the lips, eyelids and nostrils (Fig. 5.1).

Muscles of the face (Fig. 5.2)

The muscles of the face (with the exception of masseter and temporalis muscles) belong to one group and are all supplied by the VIIth (facial) cranial nerve. Typically they arise from bone and are inserted into overlying skin. They are arranged into functional groups around the openings of the

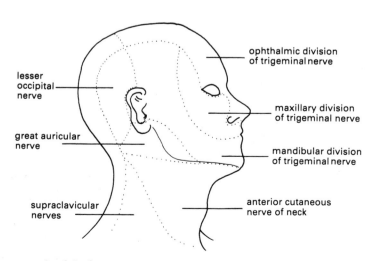

Fig. 5.1 The sensory nerve supply of the face.

A

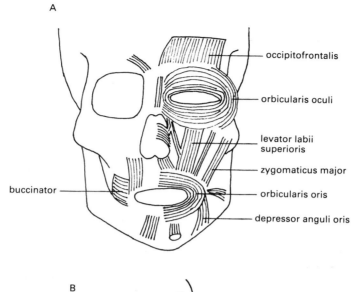

occipitofrontalis

orbicularis oculi

levator labii
superioris

zygomaticus major

orbicularis oris

buccinator

depressor anguli oris

B

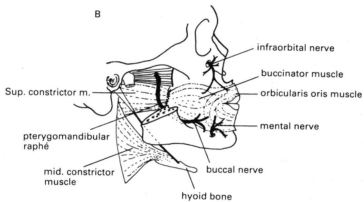

infraorbital nerve

buccinator muscle

orbicularis oris muscle

Sup. constrictor m.

mental nerve

pterygomandibular
raphé

mid. constrictor
muscle

buccal nerve

hyoid bone

C

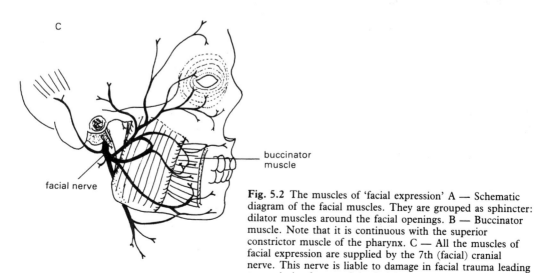

buccinator
muscle

facial nerve

Fig. 5.2 The muscles of 'facial expression' A — Schematic
diagram of the facial muscles. They are grouped as sphincter:
dilator muscles around the facial openings. B — Buccinator
muscle. Note that it is continuous with the superior
constrictor muscle of the pharynx. C — All the muscles of
facial expression are supplied by the 7th (facial) cranial
nerve. This nerve is liable to damage in facial trauma leading
to paralysis of some of the facial musculature.

head in antagonistic sphincter:dilator systems (Fig. 5.2). In man, the facial muscles around the anterior nares and external auditory meatus are of little significance, reflecting the diminished importance of the senses of smell and hearing in man.

The insertion of the facial muscles into skin produces characteristic wrinkles of the skin at right angles to their line of pull. With ageing, due to the loss of subcutaneous fat and reduced elasticity of the integument, wrinkles, for example, 'crow's feet', become more pronounced.

As a group the facial muscles are usually termed 'the muscles of facial expression'. While they are functionally important in conveying subtle changes in emotional states it should be remembered that they serve other roles. The palpebral fibres of orbicularis oculi produce blinking, thereby, with adequate lacrimal gland secretion, keeping the corneal surface moist and clean. The muscles of the lips and cheek (buccinator) are used significantly in speech and mastication. Buccinator is of particular importance in that, together with the tongue, it helps direct food between the occlusal surfaces of the teeth during mastication.

The continual activity of the facial muscles necessitates a rich nutritional supply, hence the face is highly vascular to satisfy these metabolic demands.

Arterial blood supply of the face (Fig. 5.3)

The rich blood supply of the face derives mainly from the *facial artery*. This vessel curves upward around the lower border of the body of the mandible immediately anterior to masseter muscle. The artery is readily palpable here. It then runs diagonally across the face pursuing a tortuous course as it accommodates itself to the contractions of the facial muscles it supplies.

Superior and *inferior labial* branches supply the upper and lower lips respectively. These vessels lie deep in the substance of the lips, their route being represented on the surface by the red margin of both lips. Each labial artery lies deep to orbicularis oris muscle and hence is nearer the mucosal surface of the lip than the outer (skin) surface.

The facial artery terminates at the medial corner of the eye as the *angular* artery. The artery has abundant anastomotic connections with the following arteries, which also supply the facial tissues; the *ophthalmic* artery, *transverse facial* artery and the facial artery of the opposite side. Anastomosis also occurs with the smaller arteries which accompany the terminal branches of the trigeminal nerve onto the face.

The *superficial temporal* artery exits from the upper pole of the parotid gland and crosses the zygomatic arch immediately anterior to the tragus of the ear, where it is palpable. The transverse facial artery branches from it to run forwards across the face and anastomose with the facial artery. The superficial temporal artery divides on the temple into anterior and posterior branches lying subcutaneously and can be easily observed and palpated against the dense temporal fascia.

Venous drainage of the face (Fig. 5.4)

The *anterior facial* vein commences at the medial corner of the eye by the union of the *supraorbital*, *supratrochlear* and a communicating branch with the *ophthalmic* vein. Its course across the face corresponds with that of the facial artery although lacking its tortuosity. As it passes downwards across the face the anterior facial vein receives tributaries from *infraorbital* and *mental* veins and from the *deep facial* vein which communicates with the *pterygoid venous plexus* by passing backwards deep to the ramus of the mandible.

The anterior facial vein leaves the face with the facial artery and joins with the *posterior facial* vein (retromandibular vein). The *common facial* vein so formed then enters the *internal jugular* vein.

From the above it should be noted that the anterior facial vein draining the face has venous connections via the ophthalmic vein and deep facial vein and pterygoid plexus with the *cavernous venous sinus*.

Clinical considerations

1. Tissues react to trauma whether it be mechanical, chemical, thermal or microbial in nature, by displaying an *inflammatory response*. This involves a complicated vascular and cellular reaction characterised by five cardinal signs — swelling (tumor), heat (calor), redness (rubor), pain (dolor) and loss of function of the part concerned.

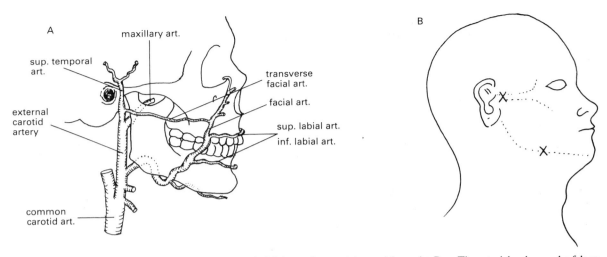

Fig. 5.3 Arterial blood supply of the face. A — The facial tissues have a rich arterial supply. B — The arterial pulse can be felt at the points marked X.

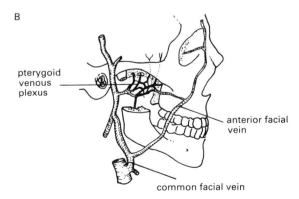

Fig. 5.4 A — Venous drainage of the face. B — The pterygoid venous plexus drains blood from the cranial, nasal and oral cavities and the facial tissues.

Due to the extreme mobility and vascularity of the facial tissues the inflammatory response is exaggerated. Oedema of the facial tissues is especially pronounced since there is a lack of dense inextensible fascia to resist swelling. Bruising following vigorous manipulation of the soft tissues during surgical procedures may be severe and extensive. Similarly, bruising may be severe following blows to the face.

2. Lacerations of the face are accompanied by profuse haemorrhage and oedema. Surgical incisions can be considered as elective lacerations and are prone to the same complications. Due to the insertion of the facial muscles into the skin of the face, wound edges can be pulled apart producing a large gaping wound, particularly if the laceration has occured perpendicular to the direction of contraction of the facial muscles. This combination of haemorrhage, oedema and the pulling apart of the edges of the wound often presents a clinical picture which appears more serious than it is in reality.

3. Rich anastomoses occur between the arteries supplying the face. If an artery is severed haemorrhage will therefore not be restricted to the proximal end of the severed vessel but will also occur from the distal segment. Haemorrhage can be controlled, depending on its site, by firm compression of the facial and superficial temporal arteries as they cross the lower border of the mandible and the root of the zygomatic arch respectively.

4. Depending on the site and depth of a facial laceration many deeper structures may be injured. Lacerations to the cheek, anterior to the parotid gland, may lead to damage of the branches of the facial nerve as they emerge from the anterior border of the gland, with resultant paralysis or paresis of the area supplied, and the parotid duct passing forwards from the gland about 1 cm below and parallel to the zygomatic arch to pierce buccinator muscle, with resultant leakage of saliva from the wound and the possibility of fistula formation.

5. Burns to the face and scalp are common, as are burns to the hands, these areas being exposed even in the fully clothed individual. Thermal or chemical burns of the face, depending on their severity and depth, produce varying degrees of skin loss and damage and result in an inflammatory response. In a superficial burn, redness (erythema) and blistering may be manifest, but deeper burns (deep partial and full thickness) will result in more widespread tissue damage. This leads to severe local oedema and plasma exudate, forming an ideal medium for the growth of pathogenic organisms resulting in widespread infection.

6. Infections of the facial tissues originating within the skin or from dental origin are potentially serious due to the ease with which they can spread through the soft tissues. Pyogenic infections in man are most commonly caused by the organisms *Staphylococcus aureus* and *Streptococcus pyogenes*. Staphylococcal infections tend to remain localised although the regional lymph nodes may become inflamed and wider spread may occur. Streptococcal infections can give rise to an extensive inflammation of subcutaneous tissues known as *cellulitis* and a spreading infection of the dermis, usually of the face, which shows a red, painful and well-demarcated lesion — *erysipelas*.

The different manifestations of infection by these two organisms is partly explained by their toxins. That secreted by the staphylococcus (coagulase) tends to promote deposition of fibrin which may help to limit its spread, and that secreted by the streptococcus (streptokinase and hyaluronidase) tends to liquify connective tissue ground substance and break down fibrin and thus promote its spread.

The lack of dense fascia which acts as a physical barrier to localise the organisms and their toxins means that infections can spread rapidly and be accompanied by marked oedema. The clinical picture of 'facial cellulitis' (as above) is frequent. If the soft tissues around the eye are involved then the oedema may be so pronounced as to close the eyelids.

7. Facial infections constitute a severe threat since, beside the phenomenon of local spread, by involving the facial veins they can spread to more distant sites. The lack of valves in the facial veins means that increased pressure in oedematous tissue may occlude the veins and retrograde drainage through venous connections will occur.

The connection between the veins of the face and the cavernous sinus via the ophthalmic veins is of critical importance. Infections can spread to the cavernous sinus and produce an infection there (cavernous sinus thrombosis) which, if unchecked, can progress to a life-threatening meningitis. Clinically, cavernous sinus thrombosis will present as dysfunction of the nerves passing forwards through the sinus principally to the orbit and face.

8. Paralysis of the VIIth cranial nerve is of either the *lower motor* or *upper motor neurone* type. The upper motor neurone type is a central lesion in the brain stem or above which is unlikely to present in dentistry but may be seen as a chance observation. The lower motor lesion may be caused by any of the factors mentioned below:

a. Transient: due to incorrect deposition of the local anaesthetic agent during inferior alveolar nerve block.
b. Trauma: from removal or spread of parotid neoplasms, laceration or penetrating injury.
c. Other: sarcoid, Bell's palsy, Ramsay-Hunt syndrome, Melkerson-Rosenthal syndrome.

The signs of facial nerve paralysis are dependent upon the site of the lesion along the course of the facial nerve.

Facial paralysis of lower motor neurone origin involves all the facial muscles of one side. One side of the face is mask-like with obliteration of the normal skin folds. This is made more apparent if the patient attempts to smile. Paralysis of buccinator muscle means that mastication is affected since food can no longer be kept between the teeth. Since orbicularis oris is affected saliva will tend to drool out from the open side of the mouth and, similarly, tears will course down the cheek from the eye due to paralysis of orbicularis oculi.

Inability to close the eyelids or blink renders the eye more liable to trauma and loss of the normal washing of the eyeball with tears by blinking means that the surface tends to become dry and more liable to infection.

6

Tongue, floor of mouth, palate, lips and cheeks

ORAL CAVITY

The oral cavity is bounded in front and at the sides by the lips and cheeks. Its roof is formed by the hard and soft palates and its base by the floor of the mouth. It contains the tongue and the teeth. The openings of the oral cavity are formed by the lips, in front, and posteriorly by the soft palate, anterior palatoglossal folds and the tongue.

The oral cavity is lined by *mucous membrane*. This is analagous to the skin. It consists of a stratified squamous epithelium (epidermis) overlying connective tissue — the *lamina propria*. Where the mucous membrane overlies the bone of the alveolar processes and the hard palate it is termed a *mucoperiosteum*.

The mucous membrane varies in colour, texture and mobility in different areas of the oral cavity. This is determined by the thickness of the epithelium, its degree of keratinisation and the firmness of the attachment to underlying structures. Surface cells are shed continually from the epithelium and are replaced by mitotic division from the basal layer. Under normal conditions this epithelial turnover is in dynamic equilibrium which may be upset in pathological states of the oral mucosa itself, or in systemic conditions.

The oral cavity is bathed continuously in *saliva* produced by the major and minor salivary glands. Saliva has cleansing and lubricant functions particularly during mastication.

Clinical considerations

1. Oral disease may be classified broadly into two categories:

a. Diseases arising in and confined to the oral cavity and its contents.
b. Systemic diseases which have *oral* manifestations.

2. The nature and course of oral diseases is influenced by the presence of a *commensal population* of micro-organisms which flourish in the warm, moist medium of the oral cavity. The commensal population is normally in stable equilibrium with the host but some of the organisms may become pathogenic if the equilibrium is upset. Thus, an *antibiotic stomatitis* may result if the composition of the commensal population is upset. The commensal fungus, *candida albicans*, is an example of an opportunistic organism which can proliferate rapidly under such conditions. Alteration in the resistance of the host can disturb the host: commensal population equilibrium and lead to infection by normally commensal organisms.

In *acute ulcerative gingivitis* reduced host resistance coupled with pre-existing tissue damage facilitates the proliferation of fusiform and spirochaete organisms in the gingival tissues of the interdental papillae.

Commensal bacteria may cause disease elsewhere in the body. *Infective endocarditis* can occur in susceptible patients who have congenital or rheumatic heart disease or who have had cardiac surgery. Oral organisms may enter the blood stream during mastication, root canal therapy, periodontal surgery or dental extraction. In the *transient bacteraemia* that is so-caused, the endocardium of susceptible patients can become infected. *Streptococcus viridans* is the oral organism commonly implicated. Appropriate antibiotic therapy prior to the dental procedure is essential.

3. *Benign* and *malignant tumours* of the oral cav-

ity can arise from any of the epithelial or connective tissues of the oral cavity. The most common malignant tumour is the *squamous cell carcinoma* which arises from the oral epithelium. Squamous cell carcinomas may arise directly from an otherwise normal epithelium or may be preceded by a *premalignant stage* in which abnormalities of the epithelium may be detected clinically and histologically.

Malignant tumours spread by direct invasion of surrounding tissues or by metastasis to distant sites. Since the lymphatic system provides a pathway for metastasis, regional lymph nodes become involved in a spreading tumour. Enlarged lymph nodes containing tumour cells are an important diagnostic sign in the detection and treatment of oral malignant disease. Systematic examination of the lymph nodes of the head and neck is essential if oral malignancy is suspected.

Oral malignancies can be treated surgically, using radiotherapy or by antimitotic drugs.

Surgical treatment, if there is lymph node involvement, usually requires a widespread excision of the lesion and surrounding normal tissue with a 'block dissection' of the neck to remove the deep cervical chain of lymph nodes. Cryosurgery is used wherever accessible lesions are present and there is no lymph node involvement, or as a palliative technique for the control of recurrences where major surgery is precluded.

Radiotherapy of oral malignancies may be complicated by *osteoradionecrosis*. The mandible, due to its relatively poor vascular supply, is particularly susceptible. The radiation causes necrosis of mandibular bone and secondary infection of the bone from teeth is likely. The existence of 'dead' bone in the mandible constitutes an area of weakness and pathological fracture may occur.

TONGUE

General considerations (Fig. 6.1)

The highly mobile tongue occupies the bulk of the oral cavity. It is a versatile organ important in speech, mastication, swallowing and as a sense organ, especially in the special sense of taste.

Essentially the tongue consists of a mass of striated muscle covered by mucous membrane. There are regional variations in the mucous membrane over its surface which give the tongue its characteristic appearance. It is normally bright pink in colour, slightly furred and velvety to the touch. This is due to the *filiform papillae*, small keratinised projections from the stratified squamous epithelium. Bright red spots on the tongue are due to the *fungiform papillae*, associated with which are found *taste buds*.

Marking the junction of the anterior two-thirds and posterior one-third of the tongue is the V-shaped *sulcus terminalis*, the apex of which points posteriorly and is marked by the depressed *foramen caecum*. Immediately anterior to the sulcus terminalis lie 7–12 *circumvallate papillae*. These consist of a large central island of tissue encircled by a deep trough. In the opposing walls of the trough taste buds are abundant. Behind the sulcus terminalis the relatively smoother mucous membrane overlies lymphoid aggregations giving the surface a slightly nodular appearance.

Over the sides and inferior surface of the tongue the mucous membrane is thin and smooth. *Foliate papillae* are found on the side of the tongue anterior to where the palatoglossal fold flows onto the side of the tongue.

Foliate papillae are usually vertical folds of mucous membrane.

The undersurface of the tongue shows several distinct features. The *lingual frenulum* is found in the midline running from the tongue to the floor of the mouth. It is a ridge of mucous membrane overlying the most superior fibres of genioglossus muscle. On either side of the frenulum the large *sublingual vein* is conspicuous under the thin mucous membrane. Lateral to this lie dark fringed folds, the *plica fimbriata*.

Glands of the tongue

Mucous glands are widely interspersed over the tongue. Aggregations of glandular tissue, both mucous and serous, are found in several sites. Serous glands open into the troughs of the circumvallate papillae, keeping them clear and unblocked by debris. In the undersurface of the tongue the anterior lingual glands (mucous and serous) are found.

Blood supply of the tongue

The continual activity of the tongue musculature necessitates a rich vascular supply which is derived from the lingual artery on both sides. The lingual artery is a branch of the external carotid artery and passes deep to hyoglossus muscle where it gives off dorsal lingual branches to the root of the tongue. After passing deep to hyoglossus muscle a sublingual branch is given off to supply the sublingual mucosa and the gingiva of the lower teeth. The main trunk of the lingual artery continues forwards deep to genioglossus to the tip of the tongue giving off a branch which lies in the lingual frenulum. There is little anastomosis between the right and left sides of the tongue except at the tip.

Venous drainage of the tongue is by branches

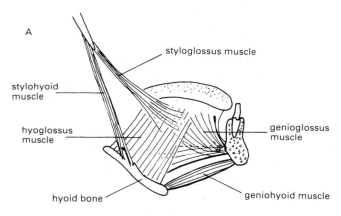

corresponding to the lingual artery. The main lingual vein drains into the internal jugular vein.

Lymphatic drainage of the tongue

The lymphatic vessels lie in a rich plexus beneath the mucous membrane of the tongue. From this plexus lymphatics drain to submental, submandibular and deep cervical lymph nodes. Two groups of nodes of the deep cervical chain are named — the *jugulodigastric* and *jugulo-omohyoid* nodes.

Lymph from the tip and undersurface of the anterior part of the tongue drains to the *submental* nodes. From here the lymph may drain *bilaterally* to deep cervical nodes.

Lymph from the sides and greater part of the dorsum of the tongue passes to the *submandibular* nodes. Alternatively, the lymphatics may pass directly to deep cervical nodes. In the median region of the tongue lymphatics may pass *bilaterally* to submandibular or deep cervical nodes.

In the most posterior portion of the tongue lymphatics drain directly to the *deep cervical* nodes.

Eventually all lymph draining the tongue will pass through some portion of the deep cervical chain and ultimately the *jugulo-omohyoid* nodes. From thence the lymphatics pass through supraclavicular nodes to enter the thoracic duct or the right lymphatic duct via the jugular trunk.

Muscles of the tongue

The muscles of the tongue, with the exception of palatoglossus muscle (see soft palate), are all supplied by the hypoglossal nerves. They can best be considered in two functional groups:

1. Muscles which alter the *shape* of the tongue, the *intrinsic* muscles.

2. Muscles which alter both *shape* and *position* of the tongue, the *extrinsic* muscles.

Of the latter group, genioglossus muscle is of particular importance in that it is the only muscle which pulls the tongue forwards. Each genioglossus muscle is fan-shaped and arises from the genial tubercles on the lingual aspect of the mandible. The uppermost fibres of these muscles pull the tip of the tongue downwards, as in the action of bringing the tip of the tongue behind the lower incisor teeth. The lower fibres of genioglossus act to pull

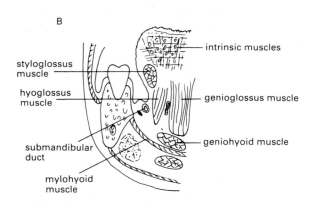

Fig. 6.1 Muscles of the tongue. A — Lateral view of tongue musculature. Note that genioglossus muscle is the *only* muscle that pulls the tongue forwards. B — Coronal section of tongue. The intrinsic and extrinsic muscles are interwoven in all three planes.

the bulk of the tongue forwards, thus allowing the tongue to be protruded out of the mouth.

Nerve supply of the tongue

The tongue develops from the first and third pharyngeal arches. Its muscles develop from occipital somites which migrate into the developing tongue carrying their motor nerve supply, the hypoglossal nerve, with them.

The sensory nerve supply of the tongue, especially towards its tip, is extremely rich. The anterior two-thirds of the tongue is supplied by the *lingual* nerve and the posterior third by the *glossopharyngeal* nerve. There is no rigid demarcation between the areas supplied by these nerves and, as elsewhere in the body, considerable overlap exists. Special sensory fibres of taste to the tongue are supplied by the lingual nerve to the anterior two-thirds and the glossopharyngeal nerve to the posterior one-third. The taste fibres associated with the lingual nerve are derived from the *chorda tympani* branch of the facial nerve which joins the lingual nerve in the infratemporal fossa.

The modalities of taste show a regional variation on the tongue. Testing of the sense of taste with suitable substances must take these variations into account.

Clinical considerations

1. Developmental disturbances of the tongue can produce congenital *microglossia* or a true *macroglossia*, due to the overdevelopment of the tongue musculature.

Secondary macroglossia can also be caused by blockage of the lymphatic drainage of the tongue, e.g. by tumour, in lymphangiomas and in hypothyroid disease. In *amyloidosis*, the accumulation of amyloid in the substance of the tongue can interfere with tongue function.

2. Alterations in the appearance of the normal tongue mucosa are relatively common. Localised atrophy of the mucosa is seen in *benign migratory glossitis* in which the atrophic patches have a disconcerting habit of wandering over the tongue mucosa.

Slight fissuring of the tongue is a normal phenomenon, e.g. median fissure. In some indi-

viduals the fissuring may be pronounced and the tongue surface can have a *scrotal appearance*. The fissures can act as a trap for oral debris and infection may result there. *Fissured tongue* is also seen as a component of the Melkerson-Rosenthal syndrome.

3. In generalised atrophy of the tongue mucosa the thinness of the epithelium produces the symptoms of *glossitis* and *glossopyrosis* and the tongue may have a red, beefy appearance. Nutritional deficiencies, particularly of the vitamin B complex, cause atrophy of the oral mucosa, of which that of the tongue is a sensitive indicator. *Vitamin B_{12} and/or folic acid deficiency* can cause severe glossitis and glossopyrosis and these may be accompanied by aphthous-type ulceration of the oral mucosa.

Iron deficiency can also cause mucosal atrophy of the tongue producing glossitis and a red, beefy tongue, although the symptoms are not as severe as with the vitamin B_{12}/folic acid deficiency.

4. *Sublingual varices.* The appearance of varices in the sublingual veins becomes more common with age. They may cause concern to patients but are harmless.

5. *Squamous cell carcinoma* of the tongue is the commonest oral malignancy. It occurs on the lateral or ventral surface of the tongue. Tumours on the dorsum of the tongue are less common.

The lesion presents as a painless mass or ulcer. Secondary infection leads eventually to severe pain. Since squamous cell carcinomas tend to metastasise through lymphatic channels, regional lymph nodes *must* be palpated to see whether infiltration by tumour has occurred.

The complicated pattern of lymphatic drainage of the tongue requires that the cervical lymph nodes must be palpated systematically on *both* sides.

FLOOR OF THE MOUTH (Fig. 6.2)

The floor of the mouth is covered by a thin mucous membrane attached laterally and anteriorly to the inner surface of the mandible where it is continuous with the mucoperiosteum of the labial gingiva. Medially the mucous membrane is continuous with the mucous membrane of the tongue forming

A

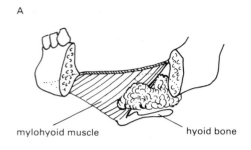

mylohyoid muscle   hyoid bone

B

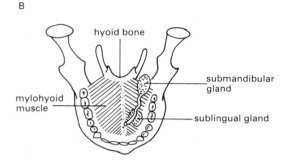

Fig. 6.2 Mylohyoid muscle. A — Lateral view. B — Plan view. Mylohyoid forms a mobile muscular diaphragm as the floor of the mouth.

a compartment between the tongue and the mandibular alveolus and teeth. This compartment is subject to great alterations in depth and shape due to the great mobility of the tongue.

When the tip of the tongue is curled back and raised firmly against the palate several distinct features can be seen. Centrally, the lingual *frenulum* — a raised ridge of mucous membrane — runs from the mandible to the tongue. The frenulum is formed by the taut upper fibres of genioglossus muscle. On either side of it are the raised sublingual papillae. These are the openings of the ducts of the submandibular salivary glands. Further back the trough between the tongue and the inner aspect of the posterior alveolus is quite deep. Palpation reveals that the sides of the trough are smooth.

The structures which lie under the mucous membrane of the floor of the mouth are supported by the mylohyoid muscles. Each muscle is attached to the mylohyoid line on the inner aspect of the mandible and converges as a thin sheet toward the midline. The more posterior fibres of each mylohyoid muscle attach to the body of the

hyoid bone. The anterior fibres meet in the midline and interdigitate with the corresponding fibres of the muscle of the opposite side. The thin muscular sheet so formed constitutes the muscular diaphragm of the floor of the mouth.

Between the upper surface of the mylohyoid diaphragm and the mucous membrane lies the sublingual compartment. Beneath the mylohyoid diaphragm, and between it and the skin surface below the chin, lies the submandibular compartment. These two compartments communicate with each other around the posterior margin of the mylohyoid muscles.

The sublingual compartment contains the geniohyoid muscles, the lingual nerve, the sublingual salivary glands and, posteriorly, part of the submandibular gland and the main duct of the submandibular gland. The duct runs forwards through the sublingual compartment to the sublingual papilla. The sublingual salivary glands lie in the anterior part of the sublingual compartment between the inner aspect of the mandible and genioglossus muscle. Unlike the submandibular gland whose ductules terminate in one major duct, the sublingual salivary gland has 10 to 20 minor ducts which open directly into the floor of the mouth.

Blood supply

The arterial blood supply of the floor of the mouth is derived mainly from the sublingual branch of the lingual artery. The sublingual artery is given off from its parent lingual artery as it ascends into the tongue along the anterior border of hyoglossus muscle. The sublingual branch passes forwards between the genioglossus muscle and the sublingual gland, which it supplies, as well as the mucous membrane of the floor of the mouth and the lingual gingival tissue. Its course in the sublingual compartment is tortuous so that it can accommodate to the movement of the region caused by the tongue and the hyoid bone.

Sensory nerve supply

Besides being the main sensory nerve of the anterior part of the tongue the lingual nerve is sensory to the mucous membrane of the floor of the mouth and the lingual gingival tissues. After traversing the infratemporal fossa the lingual nerve enters the sublingual compartment above the posterior border of mylohyoid muscle. As it enters the sublingual compartment *it lies against the inner aspect of the mandible immediately above mylohyoid muscle and just below the outer rim of the socket of the third molar tooth*. The nerve can be palpated at this site as it lies *immediately* under the mucous membrane.

From here the nerve passes sharply downwards and medially giving off branches to the lingual gingiva and the mucous membrane of the floor of the mouth. It passes under the duct of the submandibular gland and, breaking up into terminal branches, enters the muscular substance of the tongue.

Clinical considerations

1. *Dental infections* may spread from the periapical regions of the mandibular teeth into either the *sublingual* or *submandibular* compartments, depending on the relationship of the root apices of the teeth to the attachment of mylohyoid muscle to the mandible. The inflammatory response of the tissues in the compartments produces massive swelling due to the laxity and mobility of the tissues involved. The swelling may be severe enough to displace the tongue sufficient to produce difficulties in swallowing and breathing.

2. *Palpation of the submandibular duct* has to be performed *bimanually*. One hand is used extraorally to steady mylohyoid muscle. Intraorally the fingers of the other hand can be used to palpate the floor of the mouth against a steadied mylohyoid muscle. The presence of calculi or tenderness associated with the submandibular duct can be elicited.

3. *In outpatient general anaesthesia* the smooth-walled U-shaped gutter formed by the lateral border of the tongue, floor of the mouth and the inner lingual aspect of the alveolus must be 'packed-off' using a large gauze swab to prevent saliva, blood or portions of teeth from escaping into the oropharynx. In the unconscious state, such debris may pass through the larynx and enter the trachea and lungs.

4. In the *edentulous mouth* the loss of the alveolar

process results in the attachment of mylohyoid muscle to the mandible (the mylohyoid ridge) lying near the crest of the remaining alveolar bone. This varies from individual to individual. The depth of the lingual sulcus, in which the lingual flange of a denture is seated, is accordingly not great. The extent of the sulcus can be gauged by the examination of the attachment of mylohyoid muscle as it contracts during swallowing.

HARD AND SOFT PALATES

The roof of the mouth consists of the hard and soft palates bounded anteriorly and laterally by the upper dental arcade.

Hard palate

The mucous membrane of the hard palate is a *mucoperiosteum*, since it covers bone. It is tightly adherent to the underlying bone in the central region of the palate but laterally, in the angle between the bony palate and the alveolar processes, the mucous membrane is not so firmly attached. In this angle the greater palatine vessels and nerves run forwards from their foramina to supply the bulk of the mucous membrane, except for a triangular area lying behind the incisor and canine teeth as far back as the incisive papilla which is supplied by vessels and nerves reaching the palate through the incisive foramen.

Various ridges, the *palatal rugae*, are seen on the hard palate of which the centrally placed *incisive papilla* is the largest. This papilla is richly endowed with sensory nerve endings and, together with the sensitive tip of the tongue, aids in determining the consistency and nature of food particles during mastication.

The thick and keratinised epithelium of the hard palate acts in concert with the keratinised dorsal surface of the tongue as an aid to mastication.

Soft palate

The soft palate is a mobile flap lying between the naso- and oropharynx. It is attached to the free posterior edge of the hard palate and consists of a thin aponeurotic sheet into which are attached a number of paired muscles. Its free posterior border ends in a conical midline projection, the uvula. Continuous with the aponeurosis on either side are the tendons of the *tensor veli palatini* muscles. These muscles arise from the base of the skull between the pterygoid fossa and the spine of the sphenoid and sweep into the palate by hooking around the pterygoid hamuli.

The *levator veli palatini* muscles arise from the apices of the petrous temporal bones and are attached to the upper surface of the palatal aponeurosis.

Palatoglossus and *palatopharyngeus* muscles sweep downwards from the lateral parts of the soft palate to merge with the musculature of the tongue, and attach to the posterior border of the thyroid cartilage, respectively. In doing so they give rise to two vertical folds on either side of the posterior part of the oral cavity, the anterior and posterior arches of the *fauces*.

The soft palate under the actions of its associated muscles is important in controlling the exits from the nasal and oral cavities into the pharynx. Tensor veli palatini muscle tenses the soft palate. Levator veli palatini muscle pulls the tensed soft palate upwards and backwards so that it acts as a flap to close off the nasopharynx from the rest of the pharynx. Similarly, palatoglossus and palatopharyngeus muscles pull the soft palate downwards to lie against the dorsum of the tongue and seal off the oropharynx from the remainder of the pharynx.

The *uvular* muscle consists of bands of muscle attached to the posterior nasal spine which run directly backwards into the uvula.

The mucous membrane of the soft palate differs on its upper (nasal) and lower (oral) surfaces. The epithelium on the nasal surface is of the *respiratory* type while that of the oral surface is a *nonkeratinised stratified squamous* epithelium. Immediately beneath the epithelium lie aggregations of lymphoid tissue and mucous glands.

The lymphoid tissue, together with corresponding lymphoid aggregations in the posterior part of the tongue and the palatine, pharyngeal and tubal tonsils, constitutes an encircling ring of lymphoid tissue around the nasal and oral entrances to the pharynx.

The abundant mucous glands of the soft palate extend both forwards into the mucous membrane of the hard palate and downwards in the arches of the fauces to the retromolar region. Functionally, by secreting lubricating mucus, they ensure that the passage of a food bolus through the oropharyngeal isthmus during swallowing is not restricted.

The soft palate is extremely sensitive and gains its sensory nerve supply from the lesser palatine branches of the maxillary nerve.

The arterial supply to the soft palate is from the lesser palatine branches of the maxillary artery and ascending branches of the facial and lingual arteries. Venous drainage is to the pharyngeal plexus and drainage of lymph to the deep cervical chain.

Clinical considerations

1. *Fissural inclusion cysts* can arise from epithelial remnants along the lines of fusion of the embryonic processes from which the palate develops.

Nasopalatine (incisive canal) cysts are common and produce a swelling of the palate in the region of the incisive papilla.

Median palatal cysts occur in the midline of the palate and the junction of the right and left palatal processes.

2. *Failure of eruption* of canine teeth into their normal position in the dental arch can result in the teeth remaining within maxillary bone. The condition can occur bilaterally and the teeth can lie either 'outside' the dental arch, i.e. buccally, or 'inside' in the palate. Since *dentigerous cysts* can develop from the reduced enamel epithelium of unerupted or impacted teeth, clinical intervention is required.

3. '*Gag reflex*'. Stimulation of the soft palate by touching or with a foreign object initiates the 'gag reflex'. In the design of upper dentures care must be taken that the denture does not impinge onto the soft palate. During the taking of upper dental impressions, excess impression material extruding from the back of an overextended tray may cause gagging which can be extremely distressing and uncomfortable for the patient.

4. *Unilateral paralysis* of the muscles of the soft palate is a feature of *Trotter's syndrome*. This is due to a tumour of the oropharynx which, by invasion of surrounding structures, produces a set of symptoms which may be thought by patients to be of

dental origin. *Trismus* is due to the involvment of lateral pterygoid muscle. *Causalgia* and *paraesthesia* in the area of distribution of the mandibular division of the trigeminal nerve is due to tumour invading the foramen ovale. Direct involvment of the levator veli palatini and tensor palati muscles produces asymmetry and abnormal mobility of the soft palate on the affected side.

LIPS AND CHEEKS (Fig. 6.3)

The *vestibule* of the mouth is bounded laterally and anteriorly by the lips and cheeks and medially by the outer surfaces of the teeth and gingiva. The lips and cheeks form a flexible wall to the oral vestibule which can therefore be distended to accommodate food, fluid or air.

The lips and cheeks make up a muscular sheet covered on the outside by skin and on their inner surfaces by mucous membrane. Between the facial skin and the mucous membrane of the inner labial surfaces is a transitional zone — the *red margin* of the lip. Histologically the red margin represents a modified skin lacking hair follicles and sebaceous glands. The epithelium of the lip is thin and translucent accounting for the red colouration imparted by underlying blood vessels.

Buccinator muscle is the major muscle of the cheek. It is attached above to the maxilla and below to the mandible close to the line of reflection of the gingival mucoperiosteum from the alveolar processes in either case. Posteriorly it is attached to the *pterygomandibular raphe*, through which its fibres are continuous with superior constrictor muscle. Anteriorly the fibres sweep into the upper and lower lips to intermingle with the fibres of orbicularis oris.

Buccinator has an important masticatory function. Together with the tongue, the buccinator muscles aid in keeping food particles between the occlusal surfaces of the teeth during mastication.

The muscular sheet of the lip is orbicularis oris. Fibres arise from a variety of sources being continuous with those of buccinator muscle and other radial dilator muscles of the oral sphincter. Several slips of muscle arise from the *incisive fossae* of both mandible and maxilla. These muscular slips may raise ridges or *labial fraeni* on the overlying mucous membrane. In the midline pronounced labial fraeni are present, of which the upper fraenum is the largest.

Numerous mucous salivary glands are present in the lips and cheeks. The labial glands can be palpated as soft nodules between finger and thumb.

Sensory nerve supply of lips and cheeks

The upper lips receive their sensory nerve supply from the infraorbital nerves while the lower lips are supplied by the mental nerves.

Both the facial and oral surfaces of the cheek are supplied by the infraorbital nerves, the buccal branch of the mandibular division of the trigem-

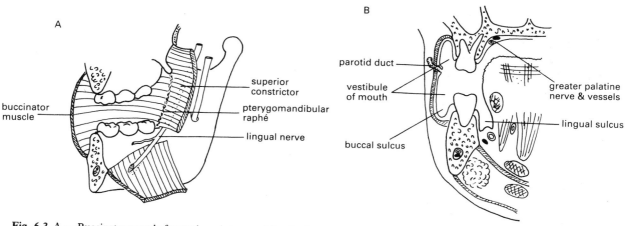

Fig. 6.3 A — Buccinator muscle forms the substance of the cheek. B — Coronal section of the oral cavity. Buccinator and the muscles of the tongue direct food between the occlusal surfaces of the teeth during mastication.

inal nerve and by the great auricular branch of the cervical plexus. The buccal nerve passes onto the outer surface of buccinator muscle from under cover of the mandible and is closely related to the external oblique line of the mandible. Its terminal branches pierce buccinator muscle to supply the mucous membrane.

Blood supply of lips and cheeks

The lips are supplied by the superior and inferior labial arteries. The arteries pass horizontally forwards from the facial artery to run deep in the substance of the lip between the orbicularis oris muscle and the oral mucosa. Their course is marked on the surface approximately by the red margin of the lip. The right and left labial arteries anastomose in the midline, a nasal branch from the superior labial artery is given off and runs upwards to the nose.

Clinical considerations

1. Trauma of the soft tissues of the lips is especially common in children, occuring as the result of falls. If the tissues have been lacerated there is pronounced bleeding and swelling. These injuries may be complicated by damage to the incisor teeth. Fragments of fractured teeth may enter the lip and are sources of infection.

2. In *dental local anaesthesia*, the numb lip may be bitten by the patient, particularly if a child. Patients and/or accompanying adults should be informed of the dangers.

3. *Mucous retention cysts* of the lower lip occur when slight trauma of the lip, such as occurs during mastication or habitual nibbling of the lip, results in the duct of one of the accessory mucous glands becoming blocked or severed. The mucous secretion accumulates in the tissues and becomes enclosed by compressed fibrous connective tissue. The mucosa of the lip becomes thin and tense as the cyst enlarges and presents as a circumscribed bluish swelling.

4. *Squamous cell carcinoma* of the lower lip is common. It presents, usually on the vermilion border, as an area of thickening, induration and ulceration or irregularity of the surface. Lip carcinomas are usually slow to metastasise and the submental and submandibular lymph nodes become involved. If the lesion is near the midline, metastasis may occur to nodes on *both* sides due to the cross-drainage of lymphatic vessels.

7

Fascial planes of the head and neck

General considerations

Connective tissue forms a general supporting matrix throughout the body. When connective tissue is differentiated and organised into fibrous, usually collagen, sheets, these are termed *fascia*.

The *superficial fascia* lies immediately beneath the skin and contains cutaneous nerves, blood vessels and lymphatics as well as varying amounts of fat. On the face the superficial fascia also contains the facial muscles.

Beneath the superficial fascia lies the *deep fascia*. These layers are separated by very loose connective tissue — areolar tissue. From the deep fascial layer extensions of fascia form fibrous septa which delineate underlying compartments which can contain muscle groups, blood vessels and/or nerves. This arrangement is seen in the limbs and in the neck. The deep fascial compartments are separated from each other by loose connective tissue. Movement between structures encased in adjacent fascial compartments is therefore not restricted. The spaces between the fascial compartments are called *fascial planes* or *spaces*. Since the fascial planes contain very loose connective tissue compared with the dense sheets of fascia bordering the planes, infections, pathological effusions and tumours can spread more easily along these planes.

Deep fascia of the neck

The neck is ensheathed in a collar of *deep fascia* (Fig. 7.1). From its deep surface fascial extensions are arranged around the viscera of the neck and the vertebral column with its associated muscle masses.

Prevertebral fascia

This layer overlies the prevertebral muscles and

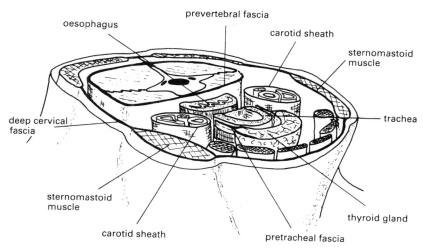

Fig. 7.1 Cross-section of neck to show the visceral, muscular and fascial compartments.

divides the vertebromuscular compartment of the neck from the visceral compartment. It is attached to the base of the skull and extends downwards into the thorax.

Pretracheal fascia

The pretracheal fascia extends from the hyoid bone downwards to the pericardium. It encloses the larynx, trachea, pharynx and oesophagus. It splits anteriorly to enclose the thyroid gland forming the gland capsule. Over the pharynx and oesophagus the fascia is not well developed and blends with the loose connective tissue in front of the prevertebral fascia. The laxity of the fascia in this area allows the pharynx to move freely and distend during swallowing. The area of loose connective tissue between the pharynx and the prevertebral fascia is called the *retropharyngeal space*. It extends from the base of the skull into the thorax.

Lateral to the pretracheal fascia as it curves backwards to enclose the pharynx is the *lateral pharyngeal space* (Fig. 7.2) which communicates behind with the retropharyngeal space.

Superiorly, where the superior constrictor muscle of the pharynx is continuous with buccinator muscle via the pterygomandibular raphé, the loose fascia lying on superior constrictor is continuous with a thin fascial layer over buccinator. This is the *buccopharyngeal fascia*. Thus the soft tissue space lying outside buccinator muscle is continuous posteriorly with the lateral pharyngeal space and laterally with the submasseteric space.

Submasseteric space

The submasseteric space lies between the *lateral surface of the mandibular ramus* and *masseter muscle* as it passes upwards to the zygomatic arch.

Submandibular spaces (Fig. 7.3)

1. The sublingual space lies between the sublingual mucosa and the upper surface of mylohyoid

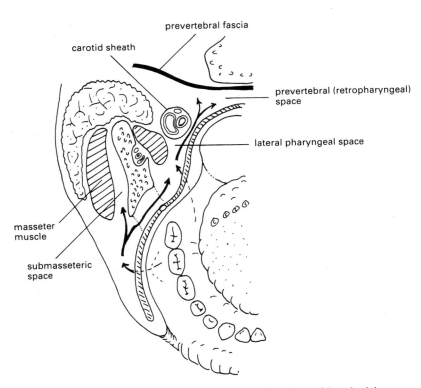

Fig. 7.2 Cross-section of head through oral cavity. The arrows indicate how infections of dental origin may spread. The retropharyngeal space communicates downwards with the mediastinum.

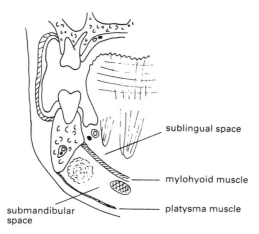

Fig. 7.3 Coronal section through oral cavity. The mylohyoid muscle separates the submandibular region into sublingual and submandibular spaces.

muscle. Laterally, it is bounded by the body of the mandible. Posteriorly, it is continuous, around the posterior border of mylohyoid muscle, with the submandibular space.

2. The submandibular space lies below the skin and superficial fascia of the submental and submandibular regions of the neck. Its depth is limited by mylohyoid muscle and it is bounded laterally by the body of the mandible. This space contains the submandibular salivary gland, submandibular and submental lymph nodes. *This space is continuous with the lateral pharyngeal space and the visceral compartments of the neck.*

Clinical considerations

Cellulitis is a diffuse inflammation of soft tissues which is not circumscribed or confined to one area. This type of reaction is in contrast to the *abscess* which is circumscribed and localised. Cellulitis occurs as a result of infection by organisms which produce *hyaluronidase* and *fibrolysins*. These can break down hyaluronic acid (the principal intercellular cement) and fibrin. Streptococci are frequent producers of hyaluronidase and are common pathogens in cellulitis.

Abscess formation in tissue spaces occurs when the infection, having entered and spread in the tissue space, becomes localised. This involves circumscribed swelling which presses on the structures adjoining the tissue space.

Infections involving specific tissue spaces

Submandibular and sublingual spaces. Diffuse infection in either the sublingual or submandibular spaces is extremely serious. The swelling produced as part of the inflammatory reaction can cause *displacement of the tongue.* This may be so marked as to produce *dysphagia* and *dyspnoea.*

Further spreading of the infection can involve both tissue spaces where displacement of the tongue becomes more pronounced. This is *Ludwig's angina.* Untreated, the cellulitis can spread down the neck under the *deep cervical fascia* to involve the *larynx* and *trachea.* Posterior spread into the *lateral* and *posterior pharyngeal spaces* can occur with the possibility of intracranial involvement. Laryngeal involvement carries the risk of oedema of the laryngeal mucosa which can severely threaten the patency of the airway.

Lateral pharyngeal space. Spread of infection into this space can occur from the submandibular and sublingual spaces or from the soft tissues of the face lying outside the *buccopharyngeal fascia.* Localisation of an infection in the lateral pharyngeal space may press on the pharynx giving *dysphagia* and even *dyspnoea.* Further spread into the *retropharyngeal space* and downwards into the *posterior mediastinum* is possible.

Submasseteric space. Infections passing backwards from the region of the cheek may pass either *deep* or *superficial* to the mandibular ramus. Those passing deep to the ramus spread into the lateral pharyngeal space (see above). Alternatively, superficial spread can occur into the submasseteric space between the masseter muscle and the ramus. The inflammatory swelling can cause severe pain and trismus due to the reflex contraction of masseter muscle.

8

The neck, pharynx and larynx

GENERAL ARRANGEMENT OF THE NECK

The skull is supported on top of the vertebral column which lies approximately in the middle of the neck. Prevertebral and postvertebral muscle masses lying in front of and behind the vertebral column are attached to the base of the skull and control its posture. The muscle masses and the vertebral column constitute the *vertebromuscular* compartment of the neck. Anterior to this lies the *visceral* compartment.

Vertebromuscular compartment

The cervical vertebral column transmits the spinal cord and its meninges. Through foramina in the transverse processes of the cervical vertebrae, the vertebral arteries pass upwards to enter the foramen magnum and aid in the formation of the arterial circle of Willis.

Cervical spinal nerves leave the spinal cord through the intervertebral foramina. The dorsal rami of the nerves course through the postvertebral muscles, supplying them, and continue as sensory nerves to the skin of the posterior aspect of the neck and scalp. The ventral rami of the cervical spinal nerves form two plexuses. The nerves C2–4 form the *cervical plexus*, while those derived from nerves C5–8 (together with the nerve from T1) form the *brachial plexus*.

Deep cervical fascia

The neck is ensheathed in a sleeve or cylinder of dense fascia which surrounds the whole neck. It is attached below to the pectoral girdle and above to the lower border of the mandible, the styloid and mastoid processes, the superior nuchal line and the external occipital protuberance. Between the angle of the mandible and the styloid process the *deep cervical fascia* splits to enclose the parotid gland and forms the capsule of the gland.

The deep cervical fascia encloses two muscles, the trapezius and the sternomastoid. Sternomastoid muscle runs obliquely upwards and backwards from the sternum and clavicle to be attached to the mastoid process and occipital bone above; on contraction it flexes the neck laterally towards its own side and turns the head so that the face is directed towards the opposite side.

Viscera of the neck

Immediately in front of the prevertebral muscles lie the major viscera of the neck.

In the midline lie the *oesophagus* and *pharynx* with the *trachea* anterior to them. Lateral to these structures lies the *carotid sheath*, a fibrous tube which contains the *carotid* arteries, *internal jugular* vein and *vagus* nerve. Interspersed along its length and in close relation to the internal jugular vein lies a chain of lymph nodes — the deep cervical nodes. The common carotid artery divides into *internal* and *external carotid* arteries at about the level of the larynx. The internal carotid artery supplies the brain and orbit while the external carotid artery supplies the face, nasal and oral cavities, most of the neck and the bone and dura mater of the neurocranium.

The thyroid gland lies in the neck closely related to the front and sides of the trachea and larynx. It consists of two large *lobes* united by a thin *isthmus* immediately in front of the upper rings of the trachea. The *parathyroid glands* are found imbedded in the upper and lower poles of the thyroid gland on either side although they may vary markedly in position from person to person.

Immediately beneath the investing deep cervical fascia in the front of the neck lie the *infrahyoid* muscles which form a sheet of muscle connecting the hyoid bone either directly with the pectoral girdle or through an intermediate connection with the thyroid cartilage. These strap-like muscles, together with the *geniohyoid* muscles which run from the inferior genial tubercles of the mandible to the hyoid bone, constitute a muscular sheet extending from the mandible to the pectoral girdle.

Sympathetic chain

Although the sympathetic outflow from the c.n.s. is restricted to the thoracic and upper lumbar segments of the spinal cord, sympathetic fibres reach the head and neck through the *cervical sympathetic chain*, an upwards extension of the thoracic chain. It lies within the posterior part of the carotid sheath and three ganglia, the *superior, middle and inferior* sympathetic ganglia, can be found along it. Postganglionic fibres from these ganglia reach their destinations by a variety of routes:

1. by joining branches of the brachial and cervical plexuses.
2. by joining branches of cranial nerves VII, IX and X distributed to structures in the head and neck.
3. by forming vascular plexuses along the subclavian, vertebral and carotid arteries.

Surface anatomy of the neck (Fig. 8.1)

Sternomastoid muscle 'divides' the neck into *anterior* and *posterior triangles* and is an important anatomical landmark which can be seen readily if the head is rotated to either side against the resistance offered by a hand held firmly against the mandible.

In the anterior triangle the *thyroid prominence* (Adam's apple) is the most distinctive feature, particularly in the male. About a centimetre above the thyroid notch the body of the hyoid bone may be palpated. Extending backwards and laterally from the midline, the remainder of the hyoid bone may be felt.

Below the thyroid cartilage lies the cricoid cartilage and the trachea. The isthmus of the thyroid

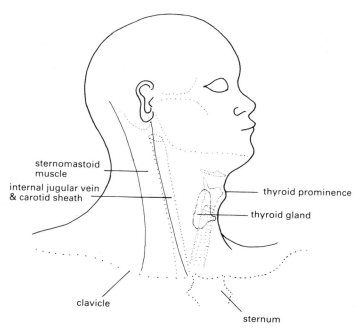

Fig. 8.1 Surface markings of the carotid sheath, internal jugular vein and thyroid gland. Sternomastoid muscle is an important anatomical landmark in the neck.

gland can be felt over the 2nd–4th tracheal rings by gently rolling it against the trachea.

The position of the carotid sheath can be marked out by a line drawn from the midpoint between the mastoid process and the angle of the jaw to the sternoclavicular joint. The carotid bifurcation lies deep to this line at about the level of the upper border of the thyroid cartilage. The carotid pulse may be palpated here and is usually visible, particularly when the neck is flexed.

The position of the deep cervical nodes (related to the internal jugular vein) is also indicated by the surface marking of the carotid sheath.

The external jugular vein descends subcutaneously over sternomastoid muscle and pierces the fascia of the posterior triangle to end in the subclavian vein. In normal circumstances the vein is barely visible but can become engorged when the central venous pressure is raised.

The cutaneous branches of the cervical plexus leave the posterior triangle and pass subcutaneously under cover of platysma muscle to supply the skin over the neck, shoulder and the upper part of the thoracic wall. The branches are (Fig. 8.2):

1. Lesser occipital nerve.
2. Great auricular nerve. This supplies the skin over the mastoid process, and the deep and superficial surfaces of the lobe of the ear. A *facial* branch supplies an area of the skin of the face in the region of the angle of the mandible.
3. Anterior cutaneous nerve of the neck. Supplies the skin of the anterior half of the neck from the lower border of the mandible to the sternum.
4. Supraclavicular nerve branches. Are sensory to the skin over the posterior triangle and the upper part of the thoracic wall.

PHARYNX (Fig. 8.3)

The pharynx is a distensible muscular tube extending downward from the base of the skull to about the level of the sixth cervical vertebra where it becomes continuous with the oesophagus. The pharynx is closely applied to the back of the facial skeleton and is continuous here with the *nasal* and *oral* cavities.

Three regions are defined in the pharynx for descriptive purposes:

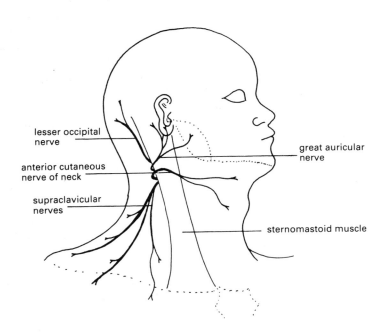

Fig. 8.2 Cutaneous branches of the cervical plexus. The great auricular nerve is sensory to facial skin over the angle of the mandible.

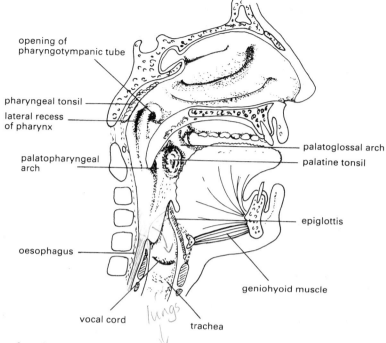

opening of
pharyngotympanic tube

pharyngeal tonsil

lateral recess
of pharynx

palatopharyngeal
arch

oesophagus

vocal cord

palatoglossal arch

palatine tonsil

epiglottis

geniohyoid muscle

lungs

trachea

Fig. 8.3 Sagittal section of nasal cavity and pharynx.

1. Nasopharynx.
2. Oropharynx.
3. Laryngopharynx.

Nasopharynx

The nasopharynx lies above the soft palate and is continuous with the oropharynx at the *pharyngeal isthmus* where the pharynx is at its narrowest. Above this, the nasopharynx is widest immediately below the base of the skull. The nasal cavities open into the pharynx through the paired *nasal choanae*. Each opening, separated by the nasal septum, extends from the base of the skull to the posterior edge of the hard palate.

Various ridges and openings are present in the lateral wall of the nasopharynx. Palatopharyngeus muscle sweeps downwards from the soft palate causing a ridge in the mucous membrane lining the pharynx which passes downwards in the wall of the oropharynx and gradually becomes less distinct. Some of the upper fibres of palatopharyngeus muscle pass horizontally backwards around the pharyngeal wall in the region of the isthmus. When the soft palate is elevated these muscle

fibres contract and produce a ridge — Passavant's ridge — against which the soft palate abuts, thereby making a more effective seal between the nasal and oral parts of the pharynx.

The *pharyngotympanic tube* opens into the lateral wall of the nasopharynx about 1.5 cm behind the inferior concha. The tube leads to the middle ear cavity and equilibrates air pressure in that cavity with that in the pharynx. The opening of the tube is surrounded by a distinct ridge which is more marked superiorly and posteriorly. Around this *tubal ridge* lies a collection of lymphoid tissue known as the *tubal tonsil*.

Immediately behind the tubal ridge the pharyngeal wall passes laterally above the upper border of superior constrictor muscle forming a deep recess or fossa. The entrance to this *pharyngeal recess* is slit-like and partially obliterated by a mucosal ridge overlying levator palati muscle.

The roof and posterior nasopharyngeal wall curve backwards overlying the base of the skull. Where the pharyngeal roof runs into the posterior wall submucosal lymphoid aggregates raise further ridges on the mucosa. These posterior lymphoid aggregates form the *pharyngeal tonsil*.

The nasopharynx is part of the respiratory tract and hence is lined by respiratory ciliated columnar epithelium.

Oropharynx

The oropharynx is common to both the respiratory and digestive tracts. Anteriorly it commences at the *palatoglossal arch* with the dorsum of the posterior part of the tongue forming a variable anterior wall. In the fold between the palatoglossal arch (which overlies palatoglossus muscle) and the palatopharyngeal ridge lies the *palatine tonsil*. The epiglottis projects upwards and backwards into the oropharynx behind the tongue from which it is separated by a central fold of tissue on either side of which lie smooth depressions — the *epiglottic vallecula*. Two further folds of tissue run downwards from both sides of the epiglottis to the arytenoid cartilages of the larynx.

Laryngopharynx

The laryngopharynx lies behind the laryngeal inlet and the posterior wall of the larynx. It is the narrowest part of the pharynx and its posterior and anterior walls are usually in contact. Two *pyriform recesses* extend forwards beside the arytenoid cartilages and the curved upper aspect of the cricoid cartilage as the larynx protrudes backwards into the pharynx.

The pharynx becomes continuous with the oesophagus at the pharyngo-oesophageal junction where the pharynx is narrowest. The junction lies opposite the lower border of the cricoid cartilage.

Muscles of the pharynx (Fig. 8.4)

The pharynx is a muscular tube which is deficient anteriorly. Three constrictor muscles make up its posterior wall and sides. They overlap each other from below upwards and have bony, cartilaginous and fibrous insertions in front. They sweep backwards, enclosing the pharynx, and insert into a median fibrous raphé which extends downwards throughout the length of the pharynx in its posterior wall from the base of the skull.

Superior constrictor muscle

The muscle arises in front from the pterygomandibular raphé and the lower part of the sharp posterior margin of the medial pterygoid plate, including the pterygoid hamulus.

The fibrous pterygomandibular raphé extends from the retromolar area of the mandible above the posterior limit of the mylohyoid line to the tip of the pterygoid hamulus. Thus superior constrictor muscle is continuous through the raphé with buccinator muscle. At its lower attachment to the raphé the lingual nerve lies *in contact* with the mandible immediately above the most posterior part of mylohyoid muscle.

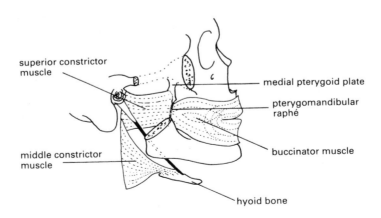

Fig. 8.4 Superior and middle constrictor muscles of the pharynx. Superior constrictor muscle is continuous with buccinator muscle through the pterygomandibular raphé.

From this extensive linear origin the muscle passes backwards enclosing the naso- and oropharynx. The upper fibres sweep upwards to be attached to the pharyngeal tubercle on the basi-occiput and the remainder of the fibres run into the median raphé in the posterior wall of the pharynx.

The muscle therefore has a free upper border extending from the pharyngeal tubercle to the medial pterygoid plate. The uppermost attachment to the posterior edge of the medial pterygoid plate is marked by a small bony spine. The wall of the nasopharynx is therefore deficient in muscle in this upper lateral region. Through this gap passes the pharyngotympanic tube and levator palati muscle. Behind this the gap extends outwards and slightly backwards as the *pharyngeal recess*. Here the wall of the pharynx consists of a sheet of fibrous tissue — the *pharyngobasilar fascia*.

Middle constrictor muscle

This muscle arises from the angle formed between the greater and lesser horns of the hyoid bone and the lower part of the stylohyoid ligament. The muscle fans out into the pharyngeal wall — the upper fibres partly overlap the lowermost fibres of superior constrictor muscle — but there is a partial gap anteriorly between the lower border of superior constrictor and the upper border of middle constrictor. Styloglossus muscle passes through the most anterior part of the gap to merge with the back and sides of the tongue. More posteriorly stylopharyngeus muscle passes downwards through the gap to be attached to the thyroid cartilage,

some of its fibres blending with the lateral pharyngeal wall.

Inferior constrictor muscle

The muscle arises from the side of the thyroid and cricoid cartilages. Its lower fibres pass horizontally around the pharynx to reach the pharyngeal raphé and overlap the oesophageal inlet. These horizontally arranged fibres are sometimes described as *cricopharyngeus* muscle and act as an oesophageal sphincter.

The majority of the muscle fibres of inferior constrictor pass upwards and backwards around the pharynx overlapping in turn middle and superior constrictor muscles. Anterolaterally there is a muscular gap in the pharyngeal wall between inferior and middle constrictor muscles. The superior laryngeal branch of the vagus passes into this gap and, after giving off the external laryngeal nerve, continues as the internal laryngeal nerve which pierces the thyrohyoid ligament to enter the larynx.

Pharyngeal plexus

This consists of a plexus of sensory and motor nerves which lie in the thin fascial covering on the external surface of the pharyngeal wall. These are derived from various sources (Table 8.1).

LARYNX

The larynx lies at the upper end of the trachea. Its opening faces backwards and slightly upwards into

Table 8.1 Sources of the pharyngeal plexus

Sensory nerve supply of pharynx	
Pharyngeal branch of maxillary division of trigeminal nerve	Roof and upper lateral wall of nasopharynx including opening of pharyngotympanic tube
Lesser palatine nerve (mandibular division of trigeminal nerve)	Mucous membrane of soft palate
Glossopharyngeal nerve	Mucous membrane of naso- and oropharynx
Vagus nerve — pharyngeal and superior laryngeal branches	Mucous membrane of oro- and laryngopharynx
Motor nerve supply of pharynx	
Glossopharyngeal nerve	Stylopharyngeus
Accessory nerve (via pharyngeal branch of vagus)	Palatopharyngeus and constrictor muscles of pharynx
Recurrent laryngeal branch of vagus	Cricopharyngeus (inferior constrictor)

the pharynx. It acts as a sphincter to regulate the entrance to the trachea and in the production of sounds.

The larynx consists of a skeletal framework of intricately shaped cartilages interconnected by ligaments, elastic membranes, synovial joints and muscles.

Laryngeal cartilages (Fig. 8.5)

Thyroid cartilage

The thyroid cartilage consists of two laminae united in front and which diverge posteriorly. Superior and inferior horns project from each lamina. The inferior horn articulates with the *cricoid cartilage* at the cricothyroid joint. Above, the thyroid cartilage is connected to the hyoid bone by the *thyrohyoid membrane*.

Epiglottis

The epiglottis is a thin leaf-like elastic cartilage attached in the midline to the inner aspect of the thyroid cartilage. It projects upwards from its attachment, lying behind the hyoid bone and the most posterior part of the tongue.

Cricoid cartilage

The ring-shaped cricoid cartilage completely encircles the airway. It is attached above to the thyroid cartilage at the cricothyroid joints and by the cricothyroid membrane. Below it is attached to the first tracheal ring by the cricotracheal membrane.

Arytenoid cartilages

The arytenoid cartilages articulate with the cricoid cartilage at its upper posterior surface. Each arytenoid cartilage is pyramidal in shape. From its base a *muscular process* projects laterally and a *vocal process* projects anteriorly.

The cricoid, thyroid and arytenoid cartilages are connected by a thin membrane, rich in elastic tissue. This is the *conus elasticus* (Fig. 8.5). It is attached to the upper border of the arch of the

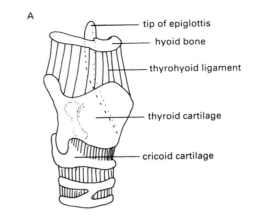

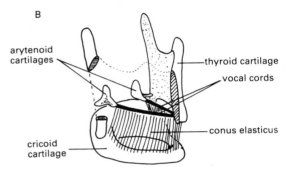

Fig. 8.5 A — Lateral view of the cartilages of the larynx. B — The arytenoid cartilages, vocal cords and conus elasticus. The rima glottidis is the space or opening between the vocal cords.

cricoid and extends upwards. The upper posterior end of the membrane is attached to the vocal process of the arytenoid cartilage and the upper anterior end to the inner aspect of the thyroid cartilage in the midline. Between these anterior and posterior attachments, the free upper border of the conus elasticus, which is thickened by longitudinal bands of elastic tissue, forms the basis of the *vocal cords*. The space between the vocal cords is the *rima glottidis*.

From the anterior borders of the arytenoid cartilages to the side of the epiglottis runs the *aryepiglottic membrane* whose thickened lower border forms the *vestibular folds* or *false cords*. Above these folds is a region of the larynx known as the *vestibule*. Between the vestibular and vocal folds is a recess, the *laryngeal ventricle*, which has a blind upward extension behind the false cords known as the *saccule*.

Movements of the cricothyroid and crico-arytenoid joints

Cricothyroid joint

The cricoid cartilage can rotate slightly backwards or forwards about a transverse axis passing through both cricothyroid joints. If the cricoid cartilage (and the associated arytenoid cartilages) rotate backwards the vocal cords will be lengthened or stretched. Forwards rotation of the cricoid cartilage will relax the vocal cords.

Crico-arytenoid joint

Each arytenoid cartilage has two types of movement relative to the cricoid cartilage (Fig. 8.6)
1. The arytenoid cartilage can *rotate* about a vertical axis.
2. The arytenoid cartilage can move laterally or medially on the cricoid cartilage.

These movements are summarised in Figure 8.6. Combinations of these movements can produce subtle alterations in the position of the vocal cords and hence in the shape and diameter of the rima glottidis. These movements are controlled by the intrinsic muscles of the larynx.

Laryngeal musculature

The movements of the larynx can be considered as:

1. Movements of the entire larynx produced by extrinsic muscles.
2. Movements within the larynx controlled by intrinsic muscles.

Action of extrinsic muscles. The larynx is suspended from the hyoid bone. Upward movements of the hyoid bone, particularly during swallowing, will move the larynx upwards aided by stylopharyngeus and palatopharyngeus muscles. This is readily demonstrated by observations and palpation of the thyroid cartilage during swallowing. Note that for this upward movement of the larynx to take place, the mandible is 'fixed' with the teeth in occlusion. Swallowing with the jaw open is possible but uncomfortable.

Action of intrinsic muscles. The intrinsic muscles of the larynx exert a protective control over the entrance to the airway by altering the position of the epiglottis and vocal cords. In addition, by altering the *position* and *tension* of the vocal cords the larynx can also produce sounds.

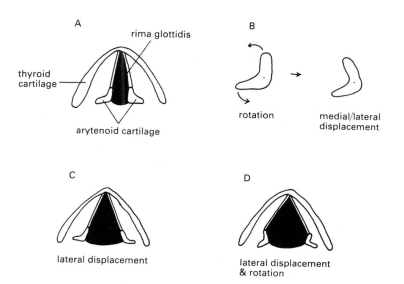

Fig. 8.6 Schematic plan views of the vocal cords and arytenoid cartilages. A — The arytenoid cartilages in quiet respiration. They are slightly abducted. B — The arytenoid cartilages can be rotated about their vertical axes or they can be displaced medially and laterally on the cricoid cartilages. C — Wide lateral displacement of the arytenoid cartilages. The laryngeal inlet is fully opened. D — Lateral displacement of the arytenoid cartilages together with rotation of the cartilages. Combination of these types of movements, together with adjustment of the tension in the vocal cords, results in the production of many different types of sounds.

Control of laryngeal inlet

When the larynx is elevated during swallowing the epiglottis is bent downwards and backwards over the laryngeal opening forming an incomplete seal. Efficient closure of the airway is accomplished by the coming together (adduction) of the vocal cords produced by muscles acting on the arytenoid cartilages (Fig. 8.6).

Interarytenoid muscles (transverse and oblique arytenoid muscles)

These muscles pass between the arytenoid cartilages. Contraction of the muscles draws the cartilages and hence the vocal cords together.

Lateral crico-arytenoid muscle

This muscle runs from the upper lateral surface of the cricoid cartilage to the muscular process of the arytenoid cartilage. Its action is to rotate the arytenoid cartilage thus moving the vocal process and attached vocal cord toward the midline and closing the airway.

Thyro-arytenoid muscle

This muscle arises from the deep surface of the thyroid cartilage near the midline and is inserted on the lateral aspect of the arytenoid cartilage. Its action is to rotate the arytenoid cartilage medially and close the vocal cords.

All the foregoing muscles are *adductors* of the vocal cords. Only one muscle abducts or opens the vocal cords. This is *posterior crico-arytenoid muscle*.

This crucial muscle arises from the posterior surface of the cricoid cartilage. Its fibres are attached to the muscular process of the arytenoid cartilage. It has two actions — its upper fibres rotate the arytenoid cartilages *laterally* and its lower fibres displace the arytenoid cartilage outwards. Both these actions *open* the vocal cords.

Cricothyroid and vocalis muscles alter the length and hence the tension of the vocal cords. Cricothyroid muscle does this by rotating the cricoid cartilage about the cricothyroid joint. Vocalis muscle consists of muscle fibres running longitudinally in the vocal cords themselves. It can therefore regulate the tension in the cords directly.

Motor nerve supply

All the intrinsic muscles of the larynx are supplied by the recurrent laryngeal nerves, with the exception of cricothyroid muscle which is supplied by a branch from the superior laryngeal branch of the vagus nerve.

The recurrent laryngeal nerves which ascend in the groove between the trachea and the oesophagus enter the larynx by passing behind the cricothyroid joint.

Blood supply

The area of the larynx above the vocal cords receives its blood supply from the superior laryngeal branch of the superior thyroid artery, the area below the vocal cords is supplied by the inferior laryngeal branch of the inferior thyroid artery.

Mucous membrane of the larynx

The larynx is lined by mucous membrane draped over the laryngeal cartilages. It has a respiratory-type epithelium (ciliated columnar) except over the vocal cords where, for functional reasons, the epithelium is stratified squamous in type.

The mucosa overlying the vocal cords has no submucosal layer and this accounts for its white avascular appearance on laryngoscopy.

The mucous membrane has a rich sensory innervation provided by the internal laryngeal nerve above the vocal cords and the recurrent laryngeal nerve below the vocal cords. These nerves are branches of the vagus nerve and are of great importance as they constitute the sensory component of the *cough reflex*.

Cough reflex

Under normal circumstances the larynx provides sufficient protection preventing material from entering the airway. If, however, this does occur the *cough reflex* provides a further protective mechanism as follows.

The cough is preceded by a deep inspiration and the vocal cords are closed tightly. A forced expiration causes a massive increase in pressure in the airway and on sudden abduction of the cords the explosive release of air into the pharynx and upper respiratory tract is usually sufficient to remove the foreign material from the airway.

Lymphatic drainage

The lymphatics of the larynx above the vocal cords drain to the upper deep cervical lymph nodes; below the cords drainage is to the lower deep cervical nodes.

Clinical considerations

1. The recurrent laryngeal nerves are closely related to the inferior thyroid arteries and may be damaged when these vessels are retracted or ligated during thyroid surgery.

The external laryngeal branch of the superior laryngeal nerve is related to the superior thyroid artery and may likewise be injured at operation.

Damage to the recurrent laryngeal nerves may be of two types:

a. Complete division — in which case the vocal cord on the injured side assumes the *paramedian* position (slightly abducted). Compensation usually occurs, the unaffected cord crossing the midline on adduction, with speech being normal or nearly normal. If both nerves suffer in this way, however, speech is lost and breathing, though possible, is difficult through the almost closed glottis.

b. Partial damage — in this case, the posterior crico-arytenoid muscle (abductor) is affected more than the adductor muscles and the cord assumes the midline position. Needless to say if the nerves are bilaterally so affected breathing is seriously impeded and tracheostomy may be necessary.

2. Cricothyroid muscle is affected in damage to the superior laryngeal nerve or its external branch leading to a loss of tension in the cord, which will have an affect on phonation by making the voice tire easily.

3. The recurrent laryngeal nerves may be involved in tumours of neck structures; thyroid gland, pharynx, oesophagus, with subsequent effects on phonation.

The left recurrent laryngeal nerve, since it descends into the thorax may also be involved in bronchial tumours, by enlarged mediastinal lymph nodes, in aneurysm of the aortic arch or by the enlarged left atrium of mitral stenosis.

4. Phonation may also be affected by local growths on the cords, either benign or malignant, resulting in hoarseness; and if the lesions are growing in size more severe disorders of phonation or breathing difficulty may result.

5. Inflammation of the mucous membrane of the larynx — *laryngitis* — can result in hoarseness or temporary loss of voice. Since the mucosa above the vocal cords is loosely attached it can swell considerably, to such an extent that the airway may be obstructed, necessitating intubation, laryngotomy or tracheostomy.

6. *Disturbances of phonation, since they can be caused by many ominous conditions must always merit detailed investigation.*

7. Laryngoscopy, directly with the laryngoscope, or indirectly by use of a laryngeal mirror, either for inspection or endotracheal intubation, is easy to perform once the long axes of the mouth, oropharynx and larynx are brought into line.

9

The temporomandibular joint

GENERAL CONSIDERATIONS

The mandible articulates bilaterally with the temporal bones at the temporomandibular joints (TMJ). These are *synovial joints* possessing a fibrous capsule enclosing the joint cavity. The fibrous capsule is lined with a highly vascular *synovial membrane* the cells of which produce the synovial fluid. Synovial fluid which contains hyaluronic acid and glycoprotein complexes is responsible for the *lubrication* of the articular surfaces of the joint and in addition has a *nutritive* function for the tissues of the articular surfaces.

Unlike the majority of the synovial joints in the body the articular surfaces of the temporal mandibular fossa and the condylar head of the mandible are not covered by hyaline cartilage. Instead, the articular surfaces are composed of a dense fibrous (collagen) articular membrane. In addition, the articular cavity is completely divided into upper and lower joint compartments by a fibrous *intra-articular disc*.

STRUCTURE OF THE TM JOINT

The mandibular condyle articulates with the squamous part of the temporal bone in a concave articular fossa — the *mandibular fossa*. The boundaries of the articular fossa are marked posteriorly by the squamotympanic fissure and medially by the articulation between the temporal bone and the greater wing of the sphenoid. The lateral boundary of the articular fossa is marked by the root of the zygomatic process of the temporal bone.

The articular fossa sweeps smoothly downwards in front to the convex *articular eminence* which is continuous laterally with the anterior root of the zygomatic process which here projects downwards as the *articular tubercle*.

The condylar head of the mandible is extremely convex anteroposteriorly and less so from side to side. The articular surface is sharply demarcated from the anterior aspect of the mandibular condyle by a bony lip. Beneath the medial two-thirds of this bony margin is the *pterygoid fossa* for the attachment of the lower part of lateral pterygoid muscle. Posteriorly, the boundary of the articular margin is indistinct. The medial and lateral poles of the condyle form relatively sharp bony protrusions. The lateral pole is palpable in the living subject during mandibular movements.

Articular capsule

The TM joint is enclosed in a fibrous articular capsule. Medially and laterally, and especially the latter, the capsule is reinforced by collagenous thickenings of the capsule forming medial and lateral ligaments.

The *lateral temporomandibular ligament* is the most important. This fibrous band runs from the *articular tubercle* on the anterior root of the zygomatic process to the lateral pole of the condyle. The collagen fibre bundles within it run downwards and backwards and are so orientated to resist backward displacement of the condylar head.

Intra-articular disc

The intra-articular disc consists of densely packed collagen fibre bundles. Posteriorly there are elastic fibres interspersed among more loosely arranged collagen fibre bundles. The disc is attached laterally and medially to the condylar poles and blends with the surrounding capsule. Posteriorly, the disc is attached, together with the articular capsule, above to the anterior margin of the squamo-tympanic fissure and below to the posterior aspect of the condylar head. The posterior region of the disc which contains the elastic tissue component has a rather looser texture than the rest of the disc. This region of the disc is much more vascular and contains sensory nerve endings of pain and proprioception.

The dense central region of the disc is relatively avascular and acellular and is not of uniform thickness, displaying anterior and posterior bands or thickenings which run from side to side. Anteriorly the disc becomes less dense. Its upper fibres attach to the anterior edge of the articular eminence and its lower fibres to the articular margin on the anterior aspect of the condylar head. Between these upper and lower extremities the collagenous fibre bundles of the disc blend with the upper fibres of lateral pterygoid muscle, becoming continuous with it. *Lateral pterygoid* muscle is therefore attached, not only to the anterior aspect of the mandibular condyle, but also to the intra-articular disc itself.

Articular surfaces

In the adult the articular surfaces of the mandibular fossa of the temporal bone and the mandibular condyle are covered by fibrous tissue — a *fibrous articular membrane*. By definition, a fibrous membrane covering bone is a periosteum, which in the TM joint is adapted to form an articular surface. Like all periostea the membrane has a potential for self-repair or remodelling. In other synovial joints the articular surface is composed of hyaline cartilage. The potential for self-repair and remodelling in hyaline articular cartilage is so severely limited as to be nonexistent.

The TM joints stand apart from other synovial joints in that remodelling of the articular surfaces is possible.

MANDIBULAR MOVEMENTS (Fig. 9.1)

Movements of the mandible are readily understood by examination of them in the living subject and

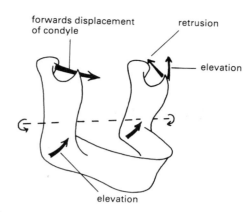

Fig. 9.1 Schematic diagram of possible movements of mandible. Downward rotation of the mandible about the axis indicated by the dotted line is a major component of mandibular opening.

comparison of these movements with similar movements re-enacted on a dried skull. First it is essential to examine the attachments and orientation of the main muscles which produce the movements. Again, these can be easily appreciated by placing plasticine models of the muscles on the dried skull.

Muscles of mastication

Lateral pterygoid muscle

This is attached to the lateral aspect of the lateral pterygoid plate and the whole of the infratemporal surface of the greater wing of the sphenoid as far lateral as the infratemporal crest. If the maxillary artery passes through the muscle on its way across the infratemporal fossa it 'splits' the muscle, giving the appearance of it arising by two separate heads. From this wide area of origin the muscle fibres pass backwards and slightly outwards to be attached to the intra-articular disc of the TM joint and the anterior aspect of the head of the mandibular condyle.

Medial pterygoid muscle

Arises from the medial aspect of the lateral pterygoid plate. A small group of fibres arise from the posterior aspect of the maxillary tuberosity and fuse with the main bulk of the muscle. The muscle passes downwards, backwards and slightly outwards to be attached to a roughened triangular area of bone lying below and behind the inferior alveolar foramen and the mylohyoid groove on the . inner aspect of the mandibular ramus.

Temporalis muscle

Is a large fan-shaped muscle which arises from the temporal fossa and also from the overlying temporal fascia. The muscle fibres in the anterior part of the muscle run almost vertically while those in the posterior part are more or less horizontal. They all converge, forming a thick tendon which passes medial to the zygomatic arch and is inserted into the apex and deep surface of the coronoid process of the mandible. The most anterior fibres are attached to the anterior surface of the mandibular ramus passing downwards to almost reach the third molar tooth.

Masseter muscle

Is attached to the lower border and deep surface of the zygomatic arch. From here the muscle passes downwards and slightly backwards to be inserted into the lateral surface of the mandibular ramus.

Resting position of the mandible

The muscles of mastication maintain the position of the mandible against gravity in the *normal resting position*. In this posture, the mandibular condyles lie in the posterior part of the articular fossa and the occlusal surfaces of the teeth are separated by a small space (2–5 mm).

Movements of the mandible (Figs 9.2, 9.3)

The intra-articular disc completely separates the joint cavity into *upper* and *lower* joint compartments.

The movements taking place within each joint compartment differ. In the *upper joint compartment* a *sliding* movement occurs between the upper surface of the disc and the articular surface of the temporal bone, whereby the intra-articular disc and mandibular condyle glide forwards onto the slope of the articular eminence.

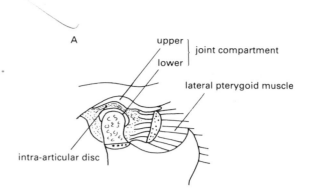

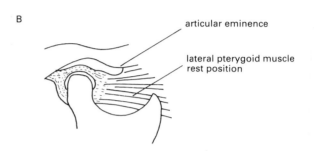

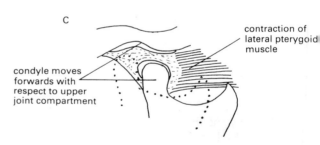

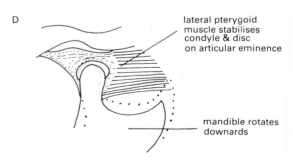

Fig. 9.2 The TM joint. A — The fibrous intra-articular disc (meniscus) is continuous with the upper fibres of lateral pterygoid muscle. B — Mandible at rest. The lower fibres of lateral pterygoid muscle are also attached to the mandibular condyle. C — Contraction of lateral pterygoid muscle pulls the disc and condyle forwards onto the articular eminence. D — Downwards rotation of the mandible completes mandibular opening.

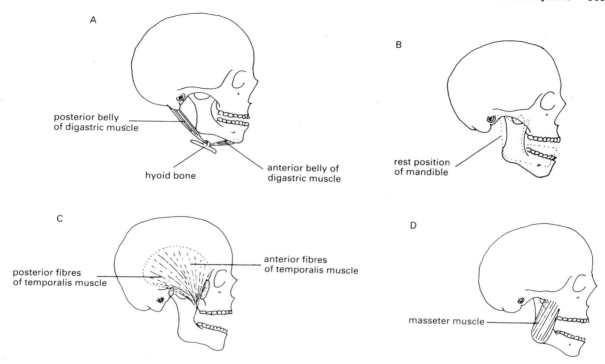

Fig. 9.3 A — Rest position of mandible. B — Contraction of digastric muscle (see A) aids in opening the mouth. C — Temporalis muscle. The anterior fibres pull the coronoid process upwards. The posterior fibres pull the coronoid process backwards. D — Masseter muscle. It is a powerful elevator of the mandible. Medial pterygoid muscle (not shown) has a similar action.

In the *lower joint compartment* movement occurs between the lower surface of the disc and the articular surface of the condyle. Since the intra-articular disc is firmly attached to the condylar poles sliding displacement between the condyle and the disc is severely limited. Instead, the predominant movement in the lower joint compartment is therefore *rotatory* as the condylar head rotates forwards relative to the intra-articular disc. The axis about which this rotation occurs is horizontal, passing through both inferior alveolar foramina (Fig. 9.1).

All mandibular movements require positional changes in both TM joints. The movements are produced by the muscles of mastication described previously and can be classified as follows:

Opening (Fig. 9.2). The lateral pterygoid muscles pull the condyle and the attached disc forwards. This movement occurs in the upper joint compartment. The medial pterygoid muscles due to their orientation will also assist in pulling the mandible forwards. The digastric muscles, acting through the stabilised pulley of a fixed hyoid bone,

aid gravity in causing the downwards rotation of the mandible, depressing the chin. This movement occurs in the lower joint compartment.

Closing. The jaw may be closed in a wide range of positions, depending on whether or not the mandibular condyle and disc are maintained in a forwards position by the contraction of lateral pterygoid muscle. This can be self-illustrated by undertaking the following three manoeuvres.

1. Open the mouth — then close the jaw so that the lower incisors 'bite' in front of the upper incisors. In this position the condyle and disc are retained in a forwards position and the closing movement has primarily involved rotation in the lower joint compartment.

2. Open the mouth — now close it so that the incisors 'bite' edge to edge. The condyle and disc are still in a forwards position due to the contraction of the lateral pterygoid muscles.

3. Open the mouth and close it normally while palpating the condylar heads bilaterally just anterior to the tragus of the ear. Compare the pos-

ition of the condyles in this normal rest position with the condyles in positions (1) and (2) above.

The masseter, medial pterygoid and temporalis muscles act to close the jaw by rotating the mandible forwards and upwards. Relaxation of lateral pterygoid is essential to allow the condyle and disc to glide posteriorly to its rest position in the articular fossa. This backwards movement is due to the contraction of the posterior fibres of temporalis muscle which run practically horizontally from their attachment toward the coronoid process. This return of the disc and condyle to the rest position is aided by the tension exerted by the elastic fibre component of the posterior part of the disc.

Protrusion

In mandibular protrusion the mandible is pushed forwards while maintaining the teeth in contact. The lateral pterygoid muscles contracting in unison pull the mandible forwards. Slight contraction of the temporalis, masseter and medial pterygoid muscles keep the teeth in contact.

Retrusion

Following mandibular protrusion the mandible is returned to its rest position by relaxation of the lateral pterygoid muscles. The posterior fibres of temporalis muscle contract pulling the mandible backwards aided by the elastic recoil of the stretched disc.

Side-to-side movements

Deviation of the mandible to any one side is effected mainly by the contraction of lateral pterygoid muscle of the other (contralateral) side. Side-to-side movements are therefore produced by alternating contractions of the lateral pterygoid muscles of each side.

Complicated combinations of all the movements outlined ensures that the mandible can occupy a myriad of positions during mastication and speech. The neuromuscular control of such a wealth of movements necessitates a vast array of sensory, proprioceptive and motor integration.

The articulation of the mandible with the base of the skull is *bilateral*. Movements occurring at one joint produce, through the rigid mandibular connection, movements at the other joint. In addition, the dental occlusion providing, as it were, another 'articulation' between the mandible and the skull, can influence TM joint movements.

The TM joints, the teeth and their supporting structures, and the muscles of mastication constitute a functional unit. Pathological changes in any constituent of this unit can thereby affect the efficiency of the unit as a whole. Thus, alterations to the dental occlusion due to the loss of teeth or the modification of the occlusal surfaces by restorative dentistry will influence the neuromuscular mechanisms controlling mandibular movements and the pattern of loading experienced by the joint tissues will also change.

These changes may not be sufficient to produce pathological alterations in the TM joints since there is a degree of physiological adaptability inherent in the neuromuscular control mechanisms. The articular membranes, within the joint, being *periostea* have, in addition, the capacity to remodel themselves to adapt to the changing loading pattern.

Mandibular posture is a useful adjunct to the muscles of the face in conveying expression. Habitual and unconscious mandibular movements can also be undertaken in various psychological states, particularly stress, depending on the individual. These movements involve *clenching* of the teeth or *grinding* of the teeth (bruxism) or a combination of both.

DEVELOPMENT OF THE TM JOINT

The TM joint develops as two cellular condensations marking the sites of the articular fossa of the temporal bone and the head of the mandibular condyle. In the intervening space a strip of densely condensed cells indicates the development of the intra-articular disc. In the region of the developing condylar head secondary cartilage develops.

The condylar cartilage is a growth cartilage playing an important role in the downwards and forwards growth of the face and it persists not only during fetal development but up to 15–20 years postnatally.

Unlike the epiphyseal growth cartilage of developing long bones, the condylar cartilage acts as an articular cartilage *and* as a growth cartilage. The articular surface of the TMJ consists of the perichondrium of the cartilage. Below this is a proliferative zone which enables the cartilage to increase the length of the ramus. The condylar cartilage gradually diminishes as growth ends becoming completely transformed into bone. The perichondrium therefore becomes a periosteum.

Growth at both TM joints increases the vertical height of the face making room for the establishment of the deciduous and permanent dentitions. Disruption of the growth activity at one TM joint may lead to asymmetrical growth of the face.

Clinical considerations

Developmental disturbances of the TM joint

1. *Condylar aplasia (failure of development).* This condition may be either *unilateral* or *bilateral* and is usually associated with abnormal development of other structures which arise from the first pharyngeal arch.

2. *Hypoplasia (underdevelopment).* Hypoplasia of the mandibular condyle is either *congenital* or *acquired.* Acquired hypoplasia is usually unilateral and secondary to a *traumatic* or *infective* insult.

These conditions interfere with the normal development and growth of the mandibular condyle and, since it plays a crucial role in the growth of the face downwards and forwards during the establishment of the *deciduous* and *permanent* dentitions, will produce *malocclusion* and *facial asymmetry.*

The extent of these will depend upon the degree of the disturbance to the joint and the age of the patient when the involvement occurred.

3. *Hyperplasia (overdevelopment).* Unilateral hyperplasia of the mandibular condyle is rare. Low-grade infection is thought to be implicated which produces an abnormal proliferative overgrowth of the condylar head resulting in a progressive elongation on the mandibular ramus and associated malocclusion.

Traumatic disturbances of the TM joint

1a. *Subluxation (partial dislocation).* In subluxation the mandibular condyle moves anteriorly over the articular eminence during opening. In this condition the joint is *hypermobile* and the subluxation can be reduced by the patients themselves.

1b. *Luxation (complete dislocation).* Complete and non-self-reducing dislocation of the mandible is more serious. It can be *unilateral* or *bilateral.* In unilateral luxation the mandible deviates to the contralateral (unaffected) side. In bilateral luxation the mouth gapes open with 'locking' of the jaw. The inability to close the mouth is hindered by contraction of temporalis, masseter and medial pterygoid muscles which, under normal circumstances, are used to close the mandible. With the condylar head *in front of the articular eminence* contraction of these muscles only serves to maintain the condylar heads in their abnormal position.

In successful treatment the condylar heads are returned to their normal position. They must therefore be moved *downwards* and *backwards* to clear the articular eminence while overcoming the contraction of temporalis, masseter and medial pterygoid muscles.

2. *Posterior dislocation.* Rarely, with severe trauma, the head of the mandibular condyle may be forced backwards and upwards through the relatively thin bone forming the articular fossa or tympanic plate so that the condylar head comes to lie in the middle cranial fossa.

3. *Fractures of the mandibular condyle.* Condylar fractures result from acute traumatic injury to the jaw, particularly a blow to the chin. The fracture tends to occur along the line of attachment of the strong lateral temporomandibular ligament.

The condylar head tends to be displaced forwards and medially due to the contraction of lateral pterygoid muscle and the mandible is deviated to the injured side by the lateral pterygoid muscle of the opposite side.

Inflammatory disturbances of the TM joint

1. *Infections.* Infections may occur as part of a generalised systemic infection or as the result of spread from adjacent regions. Retrograde infection of the mandibular ramus from the teeth may disrupt the growth of the condyle in children (see above) and in adults, depending on the severity and duration of the condition, may permanently damage the joint.

2. *Rheumatoid arthritis.* Rheumatoid arthritis is a chronic inflammatory connective tissue disease. The synovial membrane of synovial joints displays a hypertrophic synovitis. When the TM joint is involved, the inflammatory swelling produced leads to pain and tenderness of the joint with limitation of function.

Other conditions

1. *Osteoarthrosis.* Osteoarthrosis is a noninflammatory degenerative condition of joints. It is characterised by abnormal loading patterns, usually of weight-bearing joints, leading to deterioration and loss of the articular surface of joints.

Disturbances of normal mandibular movements following loss of teeth or occlusal changes after restorative procedures may produce abnormal stresses on the articular tissues of the TM joint and lead to loss of the fibrous articular membranes and thinning and perforation of the intra-articular meniscus.

2. *Ankylosis (hypomobility) of the TM joints.* Reduced mobility of the TM joint may be *unilateral* or *bilateral* and due to *intra-articular* or *extra-articular* factors. In intra-articular ankylosis the normal joint structure is replaced by fibrous or fibro-osseous tissue after an inflammatory episode following trauma or infection.

In extra-articular ankylosis there is consolidation and thickening of the tissues surrounding the condylar head and/or coronoid process.

3. *Trismus.* Trismus is an inability to open the mouth due to reflex muscle spasm. Any conditions which directly or indirectly cause increased contraction of the medial pterygoid, temporalis or masseter muscles will produce trismus e.g.

  a. Removal of wisdom teeth.
  b. Injection of local anaesthetic solutions which either directly damage muscle fibres and/or cause bleeding and haematoma formation in muscle.
  c. Fractures of the facial skeleton.
  d. Inflammation of submasseteric, infratemporal or lateral pharyngeal spaces in acute infections such as pericoronitis, tonsillitis, or parotitis.

4. *Temporomandibular joint syndrome.* In this syndrome there is a complex array of symptoms involving various degrees of trismus, craniofacial pain (which may or may not be related to the TM joints) and crepitation and/or 'clicking' of the joint either unilaterally or bilaterally. Tinnitus, and pain in the ear, neck and shoulder may also be present.

In this syndrome the complex neuromuscular mechanisms controlling mandibular posture are disrupted by a variety of factors such as occlusal disharmonies, overclosure of the mandible and bruxism/clenching. Psychological factors such as anxiety may also be present.

In this complex syndrome the abnormal or excess of normal muscle activity causes fatigue within the muscles of mastication producing pain.

Clinical examination of the TM joint

Mandibular opening

In normal mandibular opening the distance between the incisal edges is 35–45 mm.

Mandibular movements

Disorders affecting the TM joint unilaterally restrict movement on the affected side.

Palpation of the TM joint

The lateral pole of the condylar head can be palpated 1) immediately in front of the tragus of the ear and below the zygomatic arch and 2) by placing a finger in the external auditory meatus.

10

Lymphatic drainage

GENERAL CONSIDERATIONS

The lymphatic system is of great importance in the protective *immune system* of the body. It consists of three elements:

1. Aggregations of specialised cells (mainly lymphocytes).

2. A dense network of thin-walled lymphatic capillaries and interconnecting lymphatic vessels.

3. Circulating fluid — lymph, derived from tissue fluid. In lymphatics draining the intestine it contains absorbed foodstuffs, fats, amino acids, etc.

The cellular aggregations are found throughout the body as lymph nodes, in larger collections of lymphoid tissue, e.g. the palatine, lingual and pharyngeal tonsils and in specialised organs such as the thymus and spleen.

The lymphatic capillaries provide a dense drainage system for the body tissues. Tissue fluid passes readily into the lymphatic capillaries which combine to form slightly larger lymphatic vessels.

The lymphatic vessels contain many valves. Interspersed along the length of the lymphatic vessels are *lymph nodes*. Lymph enters the node capsule and percolates through the lymphoid tissue. Particulate matter may be removed from the fluid by phagocytic cells and antigenic substances can promote immunological reactions. The lymph fluid leaves the lymph node and passes along the lymphatic vessels, which usually accompany veins, to the next node and so on through a *chain of nodes*.

The flow of lymph, since there is no active pumping mechanism as in the circulation of blood, is dependent on external forces acting on the lymphatic vessels. Muscle pumping, particularly in the limbs, compresses lymphatic vessels and since they contain valves lymph flow is directed centrally.

The position of lymph nodes is not absolutely constant. In some areas the position of groups of nodes may be so constant as to be worthy of specific identification, e.g. the axillary and inguinal nodes.

Eventually the lymphatic vessels from all the body regions combine to form larger lymph ducts which discharge the lymph fluid into the venous system at the root of the neck (Fig. 10.1).

Lymph nodes of the head and neck (Fig. 10.2)

Lymph nodes are especially abundant in the head and neck. They can be considered as horizontally and vertically arranged groups of nodes of which the vertically disposed *deep cervical chain* is the most important.

Deep cervical chain (Fig. 10.2B)

The deep cervical chain extends along the internal jugular vein from the base of the skull. The lymph vessels then drain into the venous system via the right lymphatic duct or the thoracic duct.

Along the length of the chain *two* groups of nodes are identified since they lie approximately where the internal jugular vein is crossed by two muscles — the *jugulodigastric* nodes and the *jugulo-omohyoid* nodes.

The jugulodigastric nodes lie below the posterior belly of digastric muscle between the angle of the mandible and the upper anterior border of sternomastoid muscle. Jugulo-omohyoid nodes lie

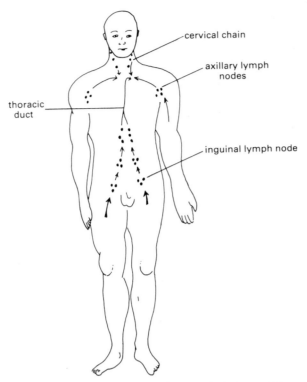

Fig. 10.1 General arrangement of lymphatic drainage of the body.

under cover of the posterior border of sternomastoid behind the internal jugular vein.

Further vertical chains of nodes extend down the neck — the superficial cervical accompanying the external jugular vein and prelaryngeal and pretracheal nodes. These chains ultimately drain into the deep cervical chain.

The horizontally disposed nodes encircle the junction of the head and neck. These are, the submental, submandibular, preauricular, mastoid and occipital nodes.

Within the oral and pharyngeal cavities an inner horizontal group of lymph nodes or lymphoid tissue is found. This consists of the palatine, lingual and pharyngeal tonsils and the tubal tonsils (at the pharyngeal opening of the pharyngotympanic tube). Isolated aggregates of lymphatic tissue are also present in the soft palate and epiglottis.

Since the flow of lymph is passively dependent on mechanical factors such as muscle pumping, lymph drainage does not always occur along predetermined routes and the patterns of lymph drainage from a specific region can be variable. In the head and neck, however, all lymph draining from the region passes ultimately along part or all of the deep cervical chain. Therefore, in clinical examination, in searching for enlarged lymph nodes (lymphadenopathy) or tender and inflamed nodes (lymphadenitis) palpation of the deep cervical chain is mandatory.

Lymphatic drainage of the oral cavity

The lymphatic drainage from the oral cavity is predominantly to the *submandibular lymph nodes*. These nodes, about three to six in number, lie between the mandible and the submandibular salivary gland. The efferent lymphatic vessels leaving the submandibular nodes pass to the deep cervical chain either running to the *jugulodigastric nodes* or joining the chain lower down in the neck at the *jugulo-omohyoid nodes*.

The submental lymph nodes lie on the surface of mylohyoid muscle behind the lower border of the mandible. They receive lymph from the skin and mucous membrane of the lower lip, the tip of the tongue and possibly from the lower teeth. Alternatively, lymph from these sites may pass to the submandibular nodes.

Efferent lymphatics leave the submental nodes and pass to the submandibular nodes or pass directly to the deep cervical chain as far down as the jugulo-omohyoid nodes.

Lymphatic drainage of the tongue (Fig. 10.2B)

The tongue has a rich lymphatic capillary plexus in the mucous membrane. The vessels draining the plexus can be considered in two groups:

1. Anterior vessels drain the anterior two-thirds of the tongue and pass to the submandibular and jugulodigastric nodes. Vessels from the tip of the tongue may pass to the submental nodes and thence to the deep cervical chain either directly or via the submandibular nodes. Lymph from the central region of the tongue may pass *bilaterally* to reach the deep cervical chain of both sides.

2. Lymph vessels from the posterior one-third of the tongue pass directly to the jugulodigastric nodes.

From the foregoing it can be seen that the fur-

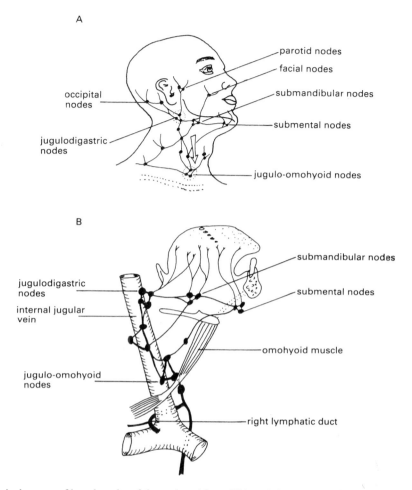

Fig. 10.2 A — Principal groups of lymph nodes of the neck and face. All lymph from the oral cavity & paraoral tissues drains eventually through the deep cervical chain. B — The deep cervical chain and the lymphatic drainage of the tongue shown for the right side. Note that there are many possible routes for lymph draining the tongue.

ther forward the origin of the lymphatic vessel from the tongue, the lower down the cervical chain may be the node in which it ends. This, together with the bilateral drainage from the posterior and central regions of the tongue, means that systematic examination of the lymph nodes draining the tongue must be *bilateral* and include the deep cervical chain *throughout its length* from mandibular to clavicle.

Lymphatic drainage of the nasal cavity and paranasal air sinuses

Lymph vessels from the mucous membrane of the anterior part of the nasal cavity pass to subman-

dibular nodes and thence to the deep cervical chain. From the posterior part of the nasal cavity lymph vessels enter the upper deep cervical chain after piercing the pharyngeal wall. The lymphatic vessels from the paranasal air sinuses follow those from the nasal cavity.

Lymphatic drainage of the teeth

Lymph vessels from the upper teeth and gums pass to either the sub-mandibular lymph nodes or posteriorly to the upper deep cervical nodes in the lateral pharyngeal space. From the lower teeth and gums, lymphatics pass to the sub-mandibular nodes and thence into the deep cervical chain.

CLINICAL CONSIDERATIONS

Cervicofacial lymph nodes may be involved in a variety of disease states which can be classified as follows:

1. Infections — local and general
2. Neoplastic disease
3. Connective tissue disease

Proliferation of lymphoid tissue within lymph nodes in any of these categories leads to *enlargement* of the node (lymphadenopathy). Enlarged nodes may also be *tender* (lymphadenitis). The occurrence of lymphadenopathy and lymphadenitis elicited by palpation is of diagnostic importance.

1. *Infections*

a. *Local infection.* Cervical lymph nodes become involved in viral and bacterial infections of the mouth, oro- and nasopharynx, ear cavities and skin of the scalp and face. Discrete groups of nodes may be involved only, e.g. the submandibular nodes and jugulodigastric nodes may be enlarged in dental abscesses.

b. *Generalised infections.* These may involve all the cervical lymph nodes as in infectious mononucleosis or rubella. Generalised constitutional symptoms will also be present.

2. *Neoplastic disease*

Lymph nodes become involved in neoplastic disease either as sites of deposition of tumour metastases from other sites or in neoplasia arising from the lymphoid tissues themselves.

Carcinomas tend to spread via the lymphatic system leading to involvement and enlargement of lymph nodes. Cervical lymph nodes become involved particularly in the spread of squamous cell carcinomas of the oral cavity and the skin of the face and scalp. Involved lymph nodes are typically 'hard' on palpation. Continued invasion of the tumour cells through the capsule of the node results in the node becoming attached or fixed to adjacent tissues.

Neoplastic disease of lymphoid series of cells produces the lymphomas and leukaemias. Lymph node involvement tends to be generalised with enlargement of cervical, axillary and inguinal groups of nodes. Enlargement of the spleen and liver also occurs (hepatomegaly and splenomegaly).

3. *Connective tissue disease*

Cervical lymph nodes may be involved in a variety of conditions in which the immune response is exaggerated and/or abnormal. In the connective tissue disorders lymph node enlargement may be present, e.g. systemic lupus erythematosus.

Examination of cervical lymph nodes

The cervical lymph nodes should be examined systematically with the palpation of occipital, facial, parotid, submental and submandibular nodes on both sides. Since all of the lymphatic vessels pass ultimately to some part of the *deep cervical chain*, this should be examined carefully. Since this is related to the *internal jugular vein*, the surface markings of this vessel provide the key to the examination of the chain.

The *jugulo-omohyoid* nodes, at the lower end of the chain, are 'hidden' behind the lower posterior border of sternomastoid muscle. On rotation of the head to the opposite side, with slight extension of the neck, this border is highlighted. Unbuttoning of the collar is essential to allow the jugulo-omohyoid nodes to be palpated.

In most instances, the enlargement of one or more of the cervicofacial lymph nodes can be explained by a local cause in the area of tissue draining to the node, e.g. dental infection, maxillary sinusitis, etc. Where an obvious cause can not be found, examination of other parts of the lymphatic system may reveal a generalised cause. The axillary and inguinal nodes and the liver and spleen should also be examined.

11

Functional anatomy: salivation, mastication, deglutition, speech

SALIVATION

Approximately 750–1500 ml of saliva is secreted per day. Saliva is a slightly viscous fluid containing water, mocupolysaccharides, immunoglobulins, an amylase and a variety of inorganic substances. Saliva acts to keep the oral cavity moist, it has a cleansing and lubricating action and is of importance in speech and, during mastication, aids in the formation of a cohesive food bolus prior to swallowing. The digestive activity of the amylase is limited since the low gastric pH inhibits amylase activity.

Saliva is secreted by *major* and *minor* salivary glands. The major glands comprise the three pairs of large salivary glands — the parotid, submandibular and sublingual glands. Minor salivary glands are found throughout the oral tissues in the lips, cheeks, tongue and hard and soft palates.

Mechanism

Salivary glands are *exocrine* glands. The secreting cells, whether mucous or serous, are highly differentiated and metabolically demanding. The secretions produced by the cells passes through ducts. In the larger glands the cells lining the ducts can modify the salivary composition by the selective removal of its constituents, particularly sodium.

The discharge of the salivary secretion into the ductal system of the glands is mediated by *myoepithelial* cells. These cells are intimately related to the glandular alveoli and small ducts and when contracted can express the salivary secretion by pressure. The myoepithelial cells are activated by

parasympathetic motor fibres — secretomotor fibres.

Parotid gland (Fig. 11.1)

The parotid gland is serous, producing a watery secretion which contains amylase. It is the largest of the salivary glands and lies in the irregular space between the ramus of the mandible and the mastoid process. Medially it is bounded by the styloid process and its associated muscles.

The superficial part of the gland overflows this space onto the face where it partly overlies masseter muscle. The gland is enclosed in a dense fibrous capsule which is derived from an upward extension of the deep cervical fascia.

Structures traversing the gland

The *facial nerve* enters the medial aspect of the gland near its posterior surface and then passes forwards lying superficially to the vascular structures which are also found in the parotid substance. The facial nerve divides into its five functional divisions within the gland and these radiate from the anterior border of the gland into the subcutaneous tissues of the face.

The *external carotid* artery enters the posteromedial surface of the gland low down and ascends through the gland substance where it divides, level with the neck of the mandibular condyle, into the *superficial temporal* and *maxillary* arteries. The superficial temporal artery crosses the root of the zygomatic arch where it may be palpated and ascends to the scalp. Before crossing the zygomatic arch it gives off the transverse facial artery which

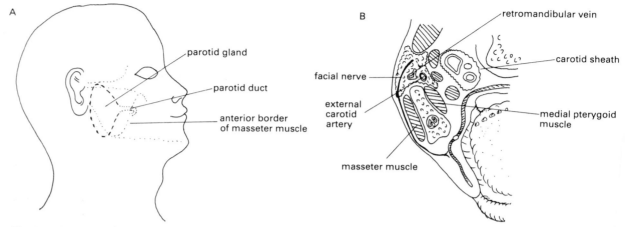

Fig. 11.1 A — Surface marking of parotid gland and its duct. B — Horizontal section of head through the parotid gland to show its relations.

runs forward through the parotid gland to leave it at its anterior border and pass forward onto the face below the zygomatic arch.

The maxillary artery passes behind the condylar neck and enters the infratemporal fossa to divide into its terminal branches which supply most of the structures of the nasal and oral cavities.

The *posterior facial* (or *retromandibular*) vein is formed within the parotid gland by the junction of the superficial temporal and maxillary veins. It descends through the gland and leaves it at its inferior border.

The *auriculotemporal nerve* (mandibular division of Vth cranial) enters the deep upper surface of the parotid gland from the infratemporal surface and leaves the gland together with the superficial temporal artery.

Parotid duct

The parotid duct leaves the anterior border of the parotid gland about one finger's breadth below the zygomatic arch. It crosses the masseter muscle and curves medially around its anterior border. It is readily palpable as it overlies the muscle, especially if the muscle is contracted when the teeth are clenched. The duct pierces the buccal pad of fat and buccinator muscle to enter the mouth where it is identifiable as a raised papilla opposite the 2nd upper molar tooth.

After the duct pierces buccinator muscle it turns forwards to run under the mucous membrane for about 5 mm before opening into the mouth. This provides a delicate valvular mechanism which prevents the retrograde passage of foodstuffs and fluids into the duct during mastication (Fig. 11.2).

Submandibular salivary gland (Fig. 11.3)

The submandibular gland is a mixed salivary gland producing a mixture of mucous and serous secretions. It consists of a larger superficial portion which is continuous around the posterior border of mylohyoid muscle with a smaller deep portion.

The superficial portion lies between the lower border of the mandible, by which it is partly covered, and digastric muscle. The deep portion of the gland continues around the posterior border of mylohyoid muscle, on which it lies. This part of the gland extends forwards under the mucous membrane of the floor of the mouth where it may reach the posterior end of the sublingual gland.

The submandibular duct begins in the superficial portion of the gland, i.e. behind and below the posterior edge of mylohyoid muscle, and curves upwards and forwards around its posterior border to pass forwards in the floor of the mouth where it opens at its narrowest point in the sub-lingual papilla. The duct is about 4–5 cm long.

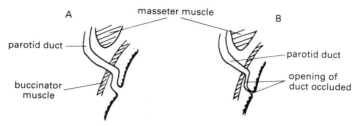

Fig. 11.2 A — The parotid duct entering the oral cavity. B — The parotid duct opening can be occluded, e.g. by foodstuffs pressing on the mucous membrane of the cheek. This acts like a valve and prevents oral contents passing in retrograde fashion into the duct.

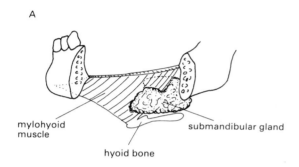

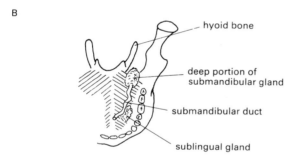

Fig. 11.3 The submandibular and sublingual glands. A — The bulk of the submandibular gland lies below mylohyoid muscle and is continuous with the deep portion of the gland around the posterior edge of the muscle. B — The submandibular duct runs forwards from the deep portion of the submandibular gland to open at the sublingual papilla. The sublingual gland opens through 10–20 small ducts directly into the floor of the mouth.

Sublingual salivary gland (Fig. 11.3)

The sublingual gland is a mixed gland in which mucous secreting acini predominate. It lies in the floor of the mouth adjacent to the inner surface of the mandible, in the incisor, canine and premolar regions. The mucous membrane overlying the gland is raised as the sublingual fold. The gland may produce a depression on the medial mandibular surface which is radiologically distinct.

Unlike the parotid and submandibular salivary glands the sublingual gland discharges its secretion through 10–20 small ducts which open directly into the floor of the mouth although a few may open into the submandibular duct.

Nervous control of salivation

Salivation is primarily controlled by parasympathetic nuclei (superior and inferior salivatory nuclei) in the brain stem. From these preganglionic parasympathetic secretomotor fibres pass to the VIIth (superior salivatory nucleus) and the IXth (inferior salivatory nucleus) cranial nerves.

VIIth cranial nerve

1. The chorda tympani branch of the facial nerve carries preganglionic parasympathetic fibres to the *submandibular* ganglion via the lingual nerve. These fibres synapse in the ganglion and postganglionic fibres leave the ganglion to various destinations:

    a. Postganglionic parasympathetic fibres pass to myoepithelial cells in the submandibular salivary gland.

    b. Postganglionic parasympathetic fibres regain the lingual nerve and are distributed via its terminal branches to the sublingual gland and the minor glands of the tongue and the floor of the mouth.

2. The greater superficial petrosal branch of the facial nerve carries preganglionic parasympathetic

fibres via a complicated route to the sphenopalatine ganglion where they synapse. Some of the postganglionic fibres from this ganglion join the greater and lesser palatine and the long sphenopalatine (incisive nerve) branches of the maxillary nerve and pass with these nerves to supply the minor salivary glands of the hard and soft palates.

IXth cranial nerve

The tympanic branch of the glossopharyngeal nerve carries preganglionic parasympathetic fibres to the tympanic plexus in the middle ear. They then join the lesser superficial petrosal nerve which again, following a complicated course, leaves the skull through the foramen ovale to the *otic ganglion* where they synapse. Postganglionic fibres join the adjacent mandibular nerve and are distributed via the *auriculotemporal nerve* to the parotid gland. Postganglionic fibres also join the inferior alveolar and buccal nerves to be distributed with their terminal branches to the mucous membrane of the cheeks and lower lip.

Sympathetic nerve supply

The high metabolic demands of the large salivary glands necessitate a rich blood supply during the production and secretion of saliva. Sympathetic vasomotor fibres from the cervical ganglia reach the salivary glands by travelling along the blood vessels which supply them.

Salivation

The parasympathetic secretomotor supply to the salivary glands is the motor component common to several reflex mechanisms which regulate the quantity and quality of saliva production.

The sensory inputs to the reflex are the smell, sight, taste and presence and texture of foodstuffs. It follows from this that there are complicated connections within the central nervous system between the sensory nuclei of the cranial nerves involved in these sensory pathways and the salivatory nuclei.

Clinical considerations

1. *Bacterial and viral infections* of the major salivary glands are the most common salivary gland diseases.

Bacterial infection occurs due to the retrograde passage of oral bacteria into the gland substance via the duct. Under normal conditions, the flow of saliva through the duct has a cleansing action. If the flow is reduced the possibility of bacterial infection increases. Salivary flow reduction occurs in debilitation and dehydration, as a side effect of some drugs and if the duct is subject to obstruction.

Mumps is an acute infectious viral disease that affects the salivary glands, especially the parotids. Where a parotitis occurs the inflammation within the gland causes a painful swelling of the gland which is resisted by the dense gland capsule.

2. *Obstruction* of the ducts of the major salivary glands may be due to trauma to the duct opening or pressure from lesions outside or within the duct. The parotid duct papilla can be traumatised opposite the second upper molar tooth by a sharp tooth cusp, badly fitting and designed denture or by a dental instrument or burr.

Salivary calculi are most commonly found in the duct of the submandibular gland. The relationship between increased salivation and meal-times produces the classical signs and symptoms of enlargement of the gland and pain prior to and during eating. Calculi can be demonstrated in the submandibular duct by *bimanual* palpation of the floor of the mouth and by radiography (Fig. 11.4).

Obstruction to the ducts of minor salivary

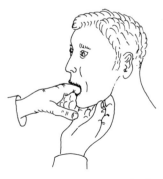

Fig. 11.4 The submandibular gland and its duct can only be palpated bimanually.

glands, particularly in the lower lip, can cause an *extravasation cyst* or *mucocoele* (see Ch. 6). Muco-coeles can also occur in the floor of the mouth. In this situation they are called *ranulae* and can interfere with tongue movements, thereby interfering with speech, swallowing and mastication.

3. The salivary glands can be involved in connective tissue disorders. In *Sjogren's syndrome* the glands, particularly the parotid, display a pronounced inflammatory lymphocytic infiltration. This is severe enough to produce swelling of the gland and to reduce salivary flow considerably. The resultant *xerostomia* is one of the triad of the syndrome, the others being a conjunctivitis and rheumatoid arthritis.

4. *Xerostomia* can also be due to a variety of causes. These include emotional and anxiety states, drug side effects, dehydration and infection of salivary glands. The dryness of the oral cavity, in which the protective and lubricating effects of saliva are reduced, prejudices the oral mucosa and fissuring, ulceration and infection of the mucosa are likely.

5. *Excessive saliva production* (sialorrhoea) is uncommon. It can occur during tooth eruption and in some cases of mental retardation.

6. *Salivary gland neoplasms.* Tumours can occur in both major and minor salivary glands although the parotid gland is most at risk. *Adenomas* occurring in the parotid gland produce swelling of the gland. The pressure exerted by the tumour may disrupt the function of the facial nerve traversing the gland and paralysis of some of the muscles of facial expression can result. Salivary gland malignancies are carcinomas of varying types. In the parotid gland, facial nerve invasion by the rapidly growing tumour produces facial paralysis. Malignant salivary gland carcinomas can also occur in the other major salivary glands and in the minor glands which are widespread throughout the oral mucosa.

MASTICATION

Mastication involves the disruption (or disintegration) of foodstuffs and the formation of a softened cohesive mass (bolus) of disintegrated food particles and saliva suitable for swallowing.

The disruption of the food is carried out between the incisal edges and occlusal surfaces of the upper and lower teeth. Complicated mandibular movements, due to the actions of the muscles of mastication, exert shearing and crushing forces on the food between the mandibular and maxillary teeth.

The incisors and canine teeth are used primarily for cutting the food into fragments of suitable size. The molar and premolar teeth, with their relatively flatter occlusal surfaces, have a grinding action. As well as controlling the *direction* of mandibular movements the muscles of mastication, particularly masseter, medial pterygoid and temporalis can vary the *compressive force* acting on the food.

During mastication it is essential that the food be continually directed between the occlusal surfaces of the teeth. This is achieved by the co-ordinated activity of the tongue, lips and cheeks. The tongue may in addition play a minor masticatory role in breaking up and moulding softer foodstuffs between its rough dorsal surface and the hard palate.

In modern urban man the consistency of the diet is softer than that of our ancestors and the forces required for complete mastication are virtually negligible. In more primitive diets, the foodstuffs require greater mastication in terms of both time and the force required. Examination of a skull used in such diets reflects these requirements. The teeth will display marked *attrition* of the occlusal surfaces. Interproximally the teeth will also be worn away due to the movement of one tooth relative to its neighbours.

The forces of mastication are transferred from the teeth to the supporting bone via the periodontal membrane. Loads applied to the facial skeleton are carried, by facial buttresses, to the neurocranium where they are dissipated. The facial skeleton can therefore be said to be designed to withstand vertical masticatory loads.

Clinical considerations

1. Untreated dental caries and periodontal disease leads inevitably to the progressive loss of natural teeth and their supporting bone. Loss of the maxillary incisor and canine teeth can alter radically an individuals appearance due to the removal of

the support for the overlying soft tissues. Besides the cosmetic considerations, the subtotal or total loss of teeth reduces masticatory function. This can be restored only partially by the provision of partial or full dentures. Since dentures are not fixed to underlying bone, their *retention* and *stability* is dependent on the provision of clasps (partial dentures only) and on varying degrees of suction and the dynamic support from the muscles of the lips, tongue and cheeks.

Maintaining a degree of masticatory efficiency with dentures requires the development of new *neuromuscular reflexes* by the muscles of mastication and those of the tongue, cheeks and lips.

SWALLOWING (DEGLUTITION)

The act of swallowing is a complicated process involving the co-ordinated activity of many muscles. It is described as occurring in stages. These are not sharply demarcated from each other since the transition from one to another occurs rapidly and smoothly.

Understanding of the process may be aided by consciously thinking of the movements of the tongue, floor of the mouth and thyroid cartilage when swallowing. In addition, palpation of the hyoid bone and thyroid cartilage helps in appreciating the large positional changes of these structures and the larynx and pharynx during swallowing.

The muscle groups active during the swallowing process are concerned with the following activities: fixation of the mandible, elevation of the hyoid bone, approximation of the tongue to the hard palate from its tip backwards, elevation of larynx and pharynx, closing of the nasopharyngeal opening and closure of the laryngeal opening.

The first stage of swallowing is *voluntary*. The mouth and teeth are closed thus fixing the mandible. A bolus, formed and shaped by the muscles of the tongue and cheeks, lies on the dorsum of the tongue. The tongue is raised and pressed against the hard palate, the movement beginning at the tip of the tongue and passing backwards. Simultaneously, the hyoid bone is elevated (by suprahyoid muscles with the mandible fixed) and pulled forwards. The bolus is propelled backwards

along the dorsal surface of the tongue and comes into contact with the tensed soft palate which helps squeeze the bolus against the tongue.

Elevation of the posterior part of the tongue propels the bolus into the *oropharynx* and the second, *involuntary*, stage commences.

The soft palate is elevated and tensed, closing off the nasopharynx. The effectiveness of the seal is enhanced by contraction of the upper fibres of superior constrictor muscle and palatopharyngeus muscle. This prevents the passage of food upwards into the nasopharynx.

The *pharynx* and *larynx* are now elevated behind the hyoid bone. Contraction of the laryngeal muscles helps pull the *epiglottis* downwards over the laryngeal opening. The bolus of food can now pass through the oropharynx, sliding over the epiglottis and aided by periodic contraction of the superior and middle pharyngeal constrictors.

In the third stage the bolus is propelled through the laryngopharynx by contractions of inferior constrictor muscle. The lowermost fibres of inferior constrictor finally relax to let the bolus enter the oesophagus.

Clinical Considerations

Dysphagia

Dysphagia is a difficulty in swallowing and most diseases of the oesophagus and its adjacent structures produce dysphagia. Dysphagia may be caused by local lesions within the wall or lumen of the oesophagus or by pressure upon it from outside. It may also be produced by other, more general, causes such as neurological disturbances, scleroderma or hysteria. As with *hoarseness*, dysphagia with solid food, lasting for two weeks or more, should be investigated promptly and thoroughly to exclude cancer of the pharynx or oesophagus.

Causes. 1. *Acute inflammation* of the mouth and pharynx may produce a short-lasting, painful dysphagia from readily apparent causes, for example, *stomatitis* or *tonsillitis*.

2. *Foreign bodies* may be swallowed accidentally or deliberately and children are particularly prone to this mishap. A foreign body may impact in the pharynx or oesophagus and result in a painful dys-

phagia. Their position is usually well localised by the patient. Foreign bodies, unless very large, irregularly shaped or sharp will usually pass into the stomach and, if so, will pass eventually, and in the main uneventfully, through the alimentary tract. If, however, they lodge in the oesophagus they will require removal because of the danger of perforation resulting in a mediastinitis.

Occasionally, an acute dysphagia results when food lodges in the oesophagus above a stricture or tumour.

3. *Congenital atresia*. The commonest maldevelopment of the oesophagus is *oesophageal atresia* with an associated *tracheo-oesophageal fistula*. Such an abnormality presents very early as a feeding difficulty with regurgitation of feed into the trachea, associated with attacks of choking, coughing and cyanosis.

Inability to pass a catheter for any distance into the oesophagus prompts the diagnosis, which is confirmed by injecting a drop of a radio-opaque medium into the blind-ended pouch and then X-raying the chest. Prompt correction and reconstruction is necessary to prevent death from aspiration pneumonia.

4. *Oesophageal stricture*. Reflux of gastric contents occurs if the cardio-oesophageal sphincter is made incompetent by a *hiatus hernia*. This results in digestion of the lower oesophageal mucosa with inflammation, ulceration, spasm, burning retrosternal or epigastric pain closely related to change of posture, and eventual stricture formation resulting in increasing dysphagia.

Reflux oesophagitis may also be produced by nasogastric intubation, repeated vomiting or the presence of gastric mucosa situated in the oesophagus.

Oesophagitis and stricture may also be caused by the ingestion, either accidentally or with suicidal intent, of strong corrosives such as caustic soda or bleach.

5. *Achalasia of the cardia* (cardiospasm). This can be defined as a neuromuscular failure of the lower oesophageal sphincter which results in progressive atony and dilatation of the oesophagus. It may be due to a failure of nerve conduction and achalasia is also seen in Chagas's disease, where the infective agent is a trypanosome. Achalasia is a predisposing factor in oesophageal carcinoma.

Dysphagia is insidious and may be associated with a feeling of retrosternal obstruction. The dilated and tortuous oesophagus fills with food and fluid which may putrify, producing halitosis, or be regurgitated, producing recurrent aspiration pneumonias.

Diagnosis is by chest X-ray, barium swallow and oesophagoscopy and treatment consists of dilatation by bouginage or cardiomyotomy. Cardiomyotomy (Heller's operation) is performed by dividing the muscle of the lower oesophagus and cardia down to the mucosa.

6. *Tumour*. Pharyngeal tumours are almost always carcinomas. They may be associated with pain in the ear (sharing a common nerve supply from the glossopharyngeal and vagus nerves) and extend into the larynx, producing hoarseness. Dysphagia occurs with weight loss, and spillover into the trachea may produce recurrent chest infections. Diagnosis is by direct examination of the pharynx, barium swallow and oesophagoscopy and treatment by radical surgery or radiotherapy, which has a poor prognosis because of lymph node involvement.

Unlike pharyngeal carcinomas, which occur more often in women at a younger age, carcinoma of the oesophagus occurs mainly in men in their later years. Its commonest site is in the midoesophagus and it is least common in the upper oesophagus. It is usually ulcerative and can extend locally to involve the circumference of the oesophagus and also invade surrounding structures and regional lymph nodes. Most are squamous cell carcinomas but occasionally adenocarcinomas are found in the lower part of the oesophagus either arising from a gastric rest or extending from the stomach.

Typically, dysphagia is of a progressive nature and occurs firstly with solid food, eventually proceeding to liquids. Associated with the dysphagia may be lymph node involvement, jaundice or hepatomegaly and the general manifestations of malignancy, for example, anaemia and weight loss.

Radiography with barium swallow may reveal a filling defect or stricture. Oesophagoscopy reveals the tumour and biopsy will confirm the diagnosis. A surgical approach with oesophagogastrectomy may be possible with tumours of the lower third of the oesophagus. Tumours above this level have a high operative mortality and supervoltage radiotherapy may be of value. Palliative treatment to relieve the dysphagia involves intubation of the oesophagus.

7. *Plummer-Vinson (Patterson-Kelly-Brown) syndrome* (sideropenic dysphagia). The dysphagia in this syndrome is associated with iron-deficiency anaemia. There is epithelial atrophy of the tongue, pharynx and oesophagus, and often the formation of a 'postcricoid web' of epithelial cells demonstrable on endoscopy or radiographically. The dysphagia may be caused by spasm at the oesophageal entrance. This condition may predispose to the development of carcinoma in the cricopharyngeal region.

8. *Pharyngeal pouch.* This diverticulum develops as a posterior protrusion of the oesophageal mucosa through a weak area between the thyropharyngeal and cricopharyngeal portions of inferior constrictor muscle. Obviously, as it enlarges, it cannot continue expanding posteriorly indefinitely and it forms into a sac that extends downwards between the oesophagus and the cervical spine to one or other side, usually the left.

Lateral displacement of the oesophagus by the sac produces a dysphagia which may be associated with regurgitation of food and bouts of inhalation pneumonia. Examination often reveals a palpable swelling in the neck which gurgles on swallowing. A barium swallow confirms the diagnosis.

Treatment is surgical, by pouch resection, combined with myotomy of cricopharyngeus muscle.

9. *Extrinsic factors,* which cause oesophageal compression, such as pressure from a retrosternal thyroid goitre, aortic aneurysm, enlargement of the heart or enlarged lymph nodes (either involved in a malignant process or one of the reticuloses) can result in dysphagia which is associated with the other signs and symptoms of the underlying cause.

Dysphagia lusoria arises from an aberrant subclavian artery which arises from the aortic arch distal to the origin of the left subclavian artery and passes across the mediastinum *behind* the oesophagus to the right upper limb. Dysphagia is present and relieved by division of the abnormal artery.

10. *Neurological disturbances,* such as single lesions of the *glossopharyngeal* and *vagus* nerves, or disorders involving the motor nuclei or upper motor neurons in the brain stem, such as *poliomyelitis* or *bulbar* and *pseudobulbar palsies,* produce dysphagia.

Occlusion of the posterior inferior cerebellar artery may result in damage to the nuclei associated with the glossopharyngeal, vagus and spinal accessory nerves, as well as other nervous structures in the area of supply, producing the *lateral medullary syndrome,* which counts dysphagia as one of its symptoms.

Diphtheria in its acute stage may produce dysphagia with the formation of an adherent membranous exudate in the pharynx. Absorption of the powerful exotoxin may affect the nervous system and give rise to the later complication of paralysis of the palate and pharyngeal muscles, causing difficulty in swallowing.

Myasthenia gravis may present with dysphagia.

11. Other causes of dysphagia include *scleroderma* and *globus hystericus,* which is not a true dysphagia and is associated with psychological stress.

ANATOMY OF SPEECH

Sounds are produced in the larynx by the passage of air through a closed glottis causing the vocal cords to vibrate. The *tension* and the *bulk,* i.e. the thickness or thinness, of the vocal cords can be varied by the intrinsic laryngeal muscles to produce sounds of differing pitch. The amplitude of the sound depends upon the rate and volume of the air passing through the larynx.

The pharynx, nasal and oral cavities above the larynx are resonating cavities which act upon the sounds produced by the larynx and modify them into the recognisable constituents of speech. The oral cavity is of particular importance as a resonator and the lips, tongue and teeth as modifiers of the initial sound produced by the larynx. Since the oral cavity is subject to remarkable variation in shape and size it is the most important source of speech sounds.

Pathological changes in the shape and size of the nasal cavity, pharynx or oral cavity, such as in the common cold, enlargement of pharyngeal or palatine tonsils, loss of teeth or in cases of cleft palate alter the normal resonating qualities of these cavities and can produce distorted speech.

12

Anatomy of anaesthesia

ANATOMY OF LOCAL ANAESTHESIA

Local anaesthetics are used in dentistry for a wide variety of surgical and conservative procedures. They are drugs which reversibly block nerve conduction when applied locally to nerve tissue in appropriate concentrations. In dentistry, they are usually administered by the following means.

Infiltration (blockage of terminal nerve branches): the injection is given directly into the area to be anaesthetised.

Regional nerve block: the injection is given into and around the nerve or nerves supplying the area involved but at a site distant from that area.

Anatomical background

The sensory nerve supply of the oral cavity is derived mainly from the maxillary and mandibular divisions of the trigeminal nerve. The maxillary division is sensory to the upper teeth, hard and soft palate, the skin and mucous membrane of the upper lip and cheek.

The mandibular division is sensory to the lower teeth and related soft tissues, mucous membrane of the anterior two-thirds of the tongue, floor of mouth, skin and mucous membrane of lower lip and cheek.

Maxillary division (Fig. 12.1)

The maxillary division leaves the cranial cavity through the foramen rotundum and enters the pterygopalatine fossa where it divides into its branches. The branches of anaesthetic importance are: infraorbital nerve, posterior superior alveolar nerve, palatine nerve, incisive (long sphenopalatine) nerve.

The *infraorbital* nerve passes forwards through the infraorbital fissure and enters a bony canal on the orbital floor. The canal opens onto the face at the infraorbital foramen where the nerve further divides into terminal labial, nasal and palpebral branches. As the infraorbital nerve passes through the infraorbital canal it may give off a *middle superior alveolar* nerve. This nerve passes laterally and downwards over the lateral wall of the maxillary sinus. Prior to the emergence of the infraorbital nerve onto the face, an *anterior superior alveolar* nerve is given off. The anterior superior alveolar nerve runs downwards and medially in the anterior wall of the maxillary sinus.

The *posterior superior alveolar* nerves (there are usually two branches) are given off from the maxillary nerve in the pterygopalatine fossa. They run down the convex posterior surface of the maxilla and enter slit-like foramina in this bone and then pass forwards and downwards in the lateral wall of the maxillary sinus to form a plexus with the terminal branches of the anterior and middle superior alveolar nerves. The superior alveolar nerves supply the maxillary teeth and the mucous membrane lining the maxillary sinus.

Infiltration anaesthesia (Fig. 12.2)

The infiltration technique is the one most commonly employed for procedures on maxillary teeth. The needle is advanced through the labial/buccal mucosa in a direction that will allow the anaesthetic solution to be deposited over the apices of the teeth involved. Since the roots of the teeth vary in length, manual palpation of the lateral surface of the maxilla can indicate the depth to which the needle should be advanced. Effective

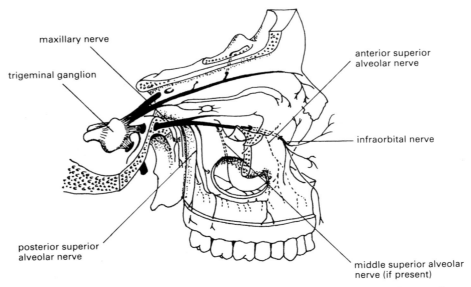

Fig. 12.1 The maxillary division of the trigeminal nerve and its branches. The middle superior alveolar nerve is present in about 50% of individuals.

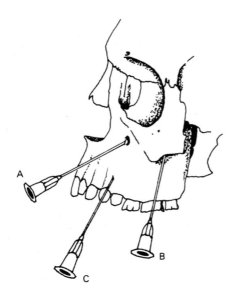

Fig. 12.2 Local anaesthesia of maxillary teeth and their supporting tissues. A — Anterior superior alveolar nerve block via the infraorbital foramen. B — Posterior superior alveolar nerve block. C — Infiltration anaesthesia through the buccal cortical plate.

anaesthesia depends on the permeation of the anaesthetic solution through the periosteum and bone of the maxilla to reach the terminal nerve branches supplying the teeth and associated gingival tissues. The bone of the maxilla overlying the

apices of the teeth is relatively thin and usually presents no serious obstacle to the infiltration of the anaesthetic.

In some individuals, however, the root of the zygomatic process may arise low down from the lateral wall of the maxilla. The resulting increased thickness of bone, related to the first and second molar teeth, may hinder the infiltration of the anaesthetic solution and reduce the effectiveness of anaesthesia. This problem can be surmounted by deposition of solution anterior and posterior to the root of the zygomatic process.

Regional block anaesthesia (Fig. 12.2)

Anterior and middle superior alveolar nerves

These nerves, supplying the incisor, canine and premolar teeth and the mesiobuccal root of the first molar, can be blocked by the deposition of anaesthetic solution into the infraorbital foramen. The infraorbital canal, when viewed from the facial aspect, passes upwards, backwards and slightly laterally. The infraorbital foramen can be readily palpated 0.5–1 cm below the inferior orbital margin on an imaginary line through the supraorbital foramen (notch), pupil of the eye and mental foramen.

Due to its upward and lateral orientation, the infraorbital canal is best approached from below and medially. The needle is advanced, intraorally, through the mucosa high in the labial vestibule in the canine region and directed toward the infraorbital foramen previously located by palpation.

In this way, effective anaesthesia of the anterior and premolar teeth, corresponding gingiva, skin and tissues of the cheek and upper lip, side of nose and lower eyelid can be attained.

Posterior superior alveolar nerve(s)

The posterior superior alveolar nerves are relatively inaccessible due to their position on the posterior surface of the maxilla. However, with powerful retraction of the cheek, a needle can be inserted behind the zygomatic process at 90° to the occlusal plane to a depth of 1–2 cm. The molar teeth and gingiva, with the exception of the mesiobuccal root of the first molar, will be anaesthetised with this procedure.

Greater palatine nerve (Fig. 12.3)

The greater palatine nerve passes onto the hard palate through the greater palatine foramen. The foramina lie at the junction of the alveolar and palatal processes of the maxilla about 3 mm anterior to the junction of the hard and soft palates, i.e. approximately in line with the junction of the second and third molar teeth. The greater palatine nerves are sensory to the mucous membrane of the hard palate with the exception of a triangular area behind the incisor teeth. The nerves run forward in the gutter between the alveolar and palatal maxillary processes. Over this region, and especially over the greater palatine foramina, the mucous membrane is not as firmly adherent to the underlying bone as elsewhere on the palate. Anaesthesia of the palatal mucosa is less traumatic if the anaesthetic solution is deposited in and around the greater palatine foramina.

Incisive (long sphenopalatine) nerve

The incisive nerves are terminal branches of the long sphenopalatine nerves which have a complicated course through the nasal cavity before en-

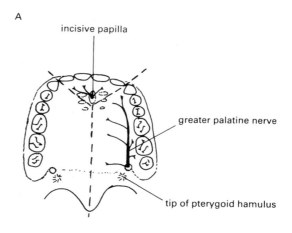

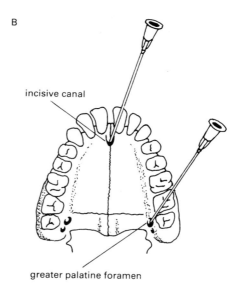

Fig. 12.3 A — Sensory nerve supply of mucous membrane and gingival tissues of the hard palate. B. — Local anaesthesia of incisive and greater palatine nerves. The mucous membrane over the incisive papilla is tightly bound to the underlying bone. In contrast, over the greater palatine foramen, the mucous membrane is much looser.

tering the mouth through the incisive canals. The nerves are sensory to the palatal mucosa behind the six anterior teeth and may also contribute sensory innervation to the maxillary incisors.

The incisive canal lies approximately beneath the incisive papilla. It passes backwards and upwards parallel to the long axis of the incisor teeth. Over the area of supply the mucosa is firmly adherent to the underlying bone. The incisive papilla has an extremely rich sensory nerve supply. Injections in this region can therefore be very painful. With correct orientation of the needle the incisive nerve can be blocked in the incisive canal.

Mandibular division (Fig. 12.4)

The trunk of the mandibular nerve (formed by union of its motor and sensory roots) emerges from the cranial cavity through the foramen ovale. It divides into *anterior* (mainly motor) and *posterior* (mainly sensory) divisions. The sensory nerves of anaesthetic importance are: buccal nerve (anterior division) lingual nerve, inferior alveolar nerve, mental and incisive nerves.

The *buccal* nerve passes forwards from the anterior division of the mandibular nerve and passes through the lateral pterygoid muscle. It runs onto the lateral surface of buccinator near its lower border from under the cover of masseter, the anterior border of the ramus of the mandible and the deep surface of the anterior border of temporalis muscle. The nerve thus crosses the upper part of the retromolar triangle at or slightly below the level of the occlusal plane. It is sensory to both the skin and mucous membrane of the greater part of the cheek.

The *lingual* nerve leaves the posterior division of the mandibular nerve deep to lateral pterygoid

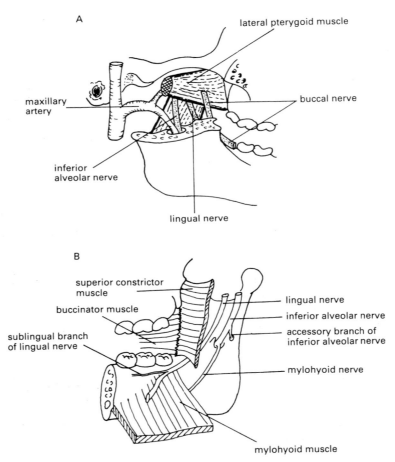

Fig. 12.4 A — Lateral view of infratemporal fossa. The buccal branch of the trigeminal nerve crosses the retromolar region immediately anterior to the mandibular ramus. B — Medial view of infratemporal fossa. The lingual nerve passes below the lower border of superior constrictor muscle to enter the oral cavity. Its sublingual branch supplies the lingual gingiva and sublingual mucous membrane. The inferior alveolar foramen lies in the centre of the ramus in the vertical and horizontal planes.

Some accessory branches of the inferior alveolar nerve may leave the main branch to enter the mandible through small accessory foramina.

muscle. It runs downwards and forwards over the lateral surface of medial pterygoid muscle and curves under the lower border of superior constrictor muscle to run forwards under the mucous membrane of the mouth. In this region it *makes contact* with the mandible on the lingual alveolar bone below and slightly behind the third molar tooth.

The nerve is sensory to the mucous membrane of the anterior two-thirds of the tongue, the floor of the mouth and lingual gingival tissues.

The *inferior alveolar* nerve arises from the posterior division of the mandibular nerve deep to lateral pterygoid muscle. It runs downwards and forwards over medial pterygoid muscle and passes into the inferior alveolar (mandibular) foramen. The nerve traverses the mandibular canal through the body of the mandible and divides terminally into a *mental* branch and *incisive* nerve branches.

The nerve is sensory to the teeth and gingiva of the lower jaw, skin of chin, lip and mucous membrane of lower lip.

The *mental* nerve is given off the inferior alveolar nerve in the mandibular canal and passes onto the face through the mental foramen. It is sensory to the skin of the chin, lower lip and corresponding mucous membrane.

Infiltration anaesthesia

The thickness and density of the outer cortical plate of the mandible restricts the use of infiltration anaesthesia to the mandibular incisors. In this region too, depending on the form of the mandibular symphysis, the thickness of the labial bony plate may reduce the effectiveness of anaesthesia.

Regional nerve block (Fig. 12.5)

Buccal nerve

The buccal nerve crosses the anterior border of the mandibular ramus in the retromolar triangle at or slightly below the level of the occlusal plane. The needle is advanced through the buccal mucosa distal to the third molar tooth and the anaesthetic solution deposited. Anaesthesia of the skin and mucous membrane of the cheek results.

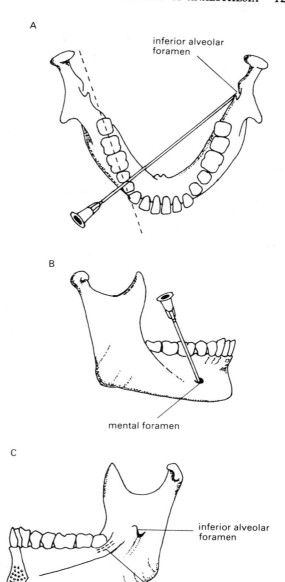

Fig. 12.5 A — Plan view of mandible during inferior alveolar nerve block. Note that the ramus diverges from the line of the dental arch (dotted line). B — Deposition of anaesthetic solution into the mental foramen. C — The lingual nerve lies in contact with the mandible below and slightly behind the third molar tooth. It is frequently anaesthetised during inferior alveolar nerve block.

Lingual nerve

The lingual nerve is usually anaesthetised during inferior alveolar nerve block.

Inferior alveolar nerve

Regional block of the inferior alveolar nerve is achieved by the deposition of anaesthetic around the nerve as it enters the canal. The mandibular foramen lies approximately in the centre of the ramus in both the vertical and horizontal axes on a level with the occlusal plane. The mandibular ramus, viewed from the front, is flared outwards posteriorly. Access to the mandibular foramen is therefore best achieved from the opposite premolar region. The needle is inserted through the mucosa slightly medial to the pterygomandibular raphé and parallel to the occlusal plane and advanced until gentle contact is made with the inner surface of the mandibular ramus. The needle is then directed posteriorly along the inner surface of the ramus until it lies adjacent to the mandibular foramen. Anaesthetic solution deposited here will result in anaesthesia of the lower teeth and gingiva and mucous membrane and skin of lower lip and chin.

Mental nerve/incisive nerve

The inferior alveolar nerve ends by dividing into a mental branch and a plexus of nerves (incisive nerve) which run forward to supply the incisor teeth. The term 'mental nerve block' is generally used to describe regional anaesthetic block for the incisor, canine and premolar teeth. Strictly speaking, however, the correct term should be an 'incisive nerve block'.

The opening of the mental foramen is directed outwards, backwards and upwards. Thus, to introduce the needle into the foramen for an incisive nerve block, the needle nust be directed downwards, forwards and inward to enter the foramen for a distance of 5 mm.

Anaesthesia of the premolar, canine and incisor teeth, skin and mucous membrane of lower lip is achieved.

Complications of local anaesthesia

Ineffective anaesthesia

1. Failure to deposit sufficient anaesthetic solution in the correct site will invariably result in incomplete anaesthesia.

2. Local anaesthetic drugs (e.g. lignocaine and procaine) are administered as weak salts and the active agent is released by ionisation in the tissues (pH 7.4). If the tissues have a lower pH, such as occurs in infections, the effectiveness of the anaesthesia may be much reduced since the ionisation of the drug and the release of the pharmacologically active agent may be inhibited.

Infection

The passage of a needle through the oral mucosa carries the attendant risk of introducing oral micro-organisms from the mucosal surface into the tissues.

Postanaesthetic trauma

Anaesthesia of the soft tissues, particularly the lips and tongue, carries with it the risk of inadvertent trauma to these tissues either during or after treatment.

Inadvertent injection into a blood vessel

The commonly used anaesthetic compounds are vasodilators. In order to prevent rapid reduction in anaesthetic concentration within the tissues most anaesthetic solutions contain a vasoconstricting agent, e.g. adrenaline tartrate used in concentrations of 1:10 000. This has a direct action on cardiac muscle and inadvertent injection of a local anaesthetic solution which contains adrenaline may cause a transient cardiac stimulation and make the patient feel mildly distressed. With the use of vasoconstrictors which have no cardiac action, e.g. noradrenaline, octapressin, this possibility may be avoided. Accidental injection into vessels may also be avoided by the use of aspirating syringes.

Intra-ligamentary anaesthesia

In this method of local anaesthesia small amounts of local anaesthetic solution are deposited within the periodontal membrane (ligament) of the tooth to be anaesthetised. The solution then 'infiltrates' down and through the periodontal membrane to reach the sensory nerve branches as they pass through the apical foramen. Anaesthesia is rapid and effective and avoids any of the problems seen with conventional infiltration anaesthesia and regional block anaesthesia. It has the potential disadvantage that the needle has to be introduced through the tissues of the gingival cuff, which may be the site of infection. Infection may therefore be spread into the periodontal membrane itself.

GENERAL ANAESTHESIA

General anaesthesia for ambulant patients is still widely used in dental surgeries. Anaesthetic drugs may be administered *intravenously* or by the *inhalation* of anaesthetic gas or gases. Frequently, the anaesthesia is *induced* by an intravenous or a gaseous agent and then *maintained* by gaseous agent(s). In some instances, short-acting intravenous agents may provide anaesthesia of sufficient duration for simple extractions.

Since the oral cavity communicates with the oropharynx, surgical procedures may interfere with the airway. Partial or total blockage of the airway, by interfering with respiration, reduces the oxygenation of the blood. If unresolved, cerebral anoxia and respiratory and cardiac arrest are inevitable. *Maintainance of the airway is therefore the critical factor during dental anaesthesia.*

During anaesthesia the normal reflex mechanisms which protect the airway are reduced or absent. The airway may be at risk from the following factors:

The tongue. In the anaesthetised state the mass of the tongue falls backwards and either totally or partially blocks the oropharynx.

Other secretions and debris. Saliva, blood, portions of teeth or intact teeth may pass from the mouth into the oropharynx. The open laryngeal inlet is unprotected by the laryngeal reflex and debris, which invariably contains oral microorganisms, can enter the trachea and/or bronchi and compromise the airway.

Vomiting: regurgitation of gastric contents may occur due to the effects of anaesthetic drugs, combined with a relaxation of the cardiac sphincter at the lower end of the oesophagus. The vomitus enters the oropharynx and can pass through the laryngeal inlet and cause a serious obstruction.

Control of the tongue and mandible

Backwards displacement of the tongue during anaesthesia can be corrected by pulling the mandible *forwards* and maintaining it in that position. This has the effect of moving the tongue forwards by pulling on the relaxed genioglossus muscle. (In the unanaesthetised state, this muscle is the *only* muscle which can move the tongue forwards.)

Mobility of the mandible in anaesthesia is enhanced by relaxation of the muscles of mastication. Downwards pressure on the mandible during extraction, combined with forwards pressure to keep the tongue from obstructing the airway, can cause the mandibular condyles to disengage from the mandibular fossae, resulting in a *dislocation*. This must be checked for and corrected before the anaesthesia is terminated and normal muscle tone and control has returned.

Control of the passage of oral debris

The danger of the passage of oral debris into the oropharynx can be substantially decreased by the use of *gauze packs*. These are placed to seal off the entrance to the oropharynx, particularly the smooth gutter lying between the side of the tongue and the mandibular alveolus. As well as preventing the movement of debris, saliva and blood, the pack also has the effect of promoting *nasal respiration*, which is critical if the anaesthesia is being maintained by an anaesthetic gas delivered via a nasal mask.

Haemorrhage from extraction sites is copious in general anaesthesia compared to similar extractions carried out under local anaesthesia which contain *vasoconstrictors*.

Control of vomiting

Vomiting under anaesthesia can be avoided if the stomach is empty. Patients undergoing anaesthesia should be given firm instructions not to take food or fluids for at least four hours before the anaesthetic.

13

Anatomy of intravenous and intramuscular injection

INTRAVENOUS INJECTION (Fig. 13.1)

Injections of hypnotic or sedative drugs as well as general anaesthetic agents are performed via the intravenous route. Phlebotomy is also performed by venepuncture. The common site for these procedures lies anterior to the elbow joint in the *cubital fossa*.

The cubital fossa is triangular with its base lying between the humeral epicondyles and its medial and lateral borders formed by the pronator teres and brachioradialis muscles, respectively. The capsule of the elbow joint is overlain by brachialis and supinator muscles forming the floor of the fossa and these in their turn are overlain by the contents of the fossa; namely, the median nerve, the brachial artery, the tendon of biceps muscle and the radial nerve, from medial to lateral. These structures are surrounded by fat and roofed in by the deep fascia of the forearm strengthened medially by the *bicipital aponeurosis* which lies over the brachial artery and the median nerve.

Lying subcutaneously on the deep fascia are, laterally, the *cephalic vein*, which runs from the anatomical 'snuff-box' up the lateral side of the forearm, lies anterior to the cubital fossa and then lateral to biceps muscle, and, medially, the *basilic vein*, which runs up the posteromedial side of the forearm, passes anterior to the cubital fossa and then lies medial to biceps muscle.

Joining these two veins across the front of the cubital fossa is the prominent *median cubital vein* and it is this vein that is commonly chosen for venepuncture and intravenous injection. The bicipital aponeurosis lies deep to it and protects the brachial artery and the median nerve from injury but, even so, damage to these structures and, oc-

casionally, to a superficial, aberrant, ulnar artery may still occur.

In view of this, intravenous injections of irritant substances, e.g. anaesthetic drugs, tend to be given into the veins on the dorsum of the hand or into the cubital vein proximal to the wrist. Injections of this type are usually given through previously sited intravenous cannulae through which further doses of the same or other substances may be given without recourse to further venepuncture.

Intravenous infusions are given through cannulae which should be sited away from either the elbow or wrist joints so that the position of the cannula is not compromised during movements of these joints.

In cases of shock with collapse of the superficial veins an emergency 'cut-down' may be performed on the cubital vein, which is fairly constant in its position at the wrist, lying just posterior to the *styloid process* of the radius.

INTRAMUSCULAR INJECTIONS (Fig. 13.2)

Intramuscular injections are least painful when given into a large muscle mass and the gluteal muscles of the buttock are therefore a very common site for this procedure. However, a misplaced injection into this area may damage the large *sciatic nerve* as it passes through the buttock from the *greater sciatic notch* to the posterior (hamstring) compartment of the thigh.

An outwardly curving line drawn between a point midway between the *posterior superior iliac spine* and the *ischial tuberosity* and a point midway between the ischial tuberosity and the *greater trochanter* of the femur represents the surface mark-

A

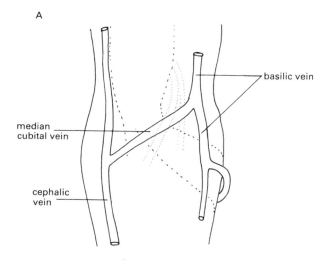

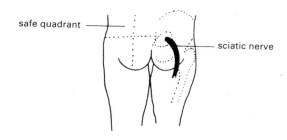

Fig. 13.2 Diagrammatic view of buttocks. The upper outer quadrant of the buttock is the safest site for intramuscular injection.

B

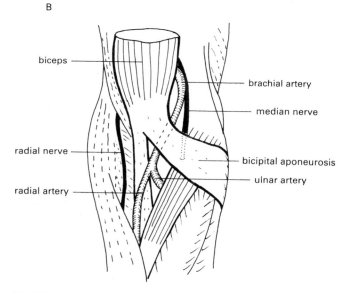

Fig. 13.1 Anatomy of the cubital fossa. A — Cubital fossa of the right arm. The superficial veins crossing the fossa are accessible for intravenous injection and phlebotomy. The median cubital vein is commonly chosen. B — Deeper structures of cubital fossa of right arm. The brachial artery and median nerve are separated from the median cubital vein by the bicipital aponeurosis.

ing of this nerve, and intramuscular injections should be given away from this area. It is standard practice to mentally divide the buttock by means of a vertical and a horizontal line into four quadrants and to place intramuscular injections into the *upper outer quadrant* to prevent inadvertent damage to the nerve.

14

Embryology of the face, nasal and oral cavities

EMBRYOLOGY

The oral cavity, nasal cavities and face develop rapidly from the fourth week of intrauterine life so that, by the eighth week, the embryo is recognisably human.

At the beginning of the fourth week the cranial end of the embryo is dominated by the large *forebrain* swelling. This is separated from the *pericardial* swelling by an intervening slit which makes the entrance to a blind cavity — the *stomatodeum*. This stomatodeum (buccal) cavity is separated from the pharyngeal end of the foregut by the thin *buccopharyngeal membrane* which ruptures during the fourth week linking the primitive oral cavity with the foregut.

DEVELOPMENT OF THE PHARYNX AND PHARYNGEAL ARCHES (Fig. 14.1)

The developing pharynx is lined by *endoderm* which grows outwards into the surrounding mesoderm in the fourth and fifth weeks to form the *pharyngeal pouches* along the lateral walls of the pharynx. At the same time *pharyngeal (branchial) clefts* appear on the outer aspect of the pharyngeal wall corresponding to the pouches. The mesoderm which is pushed aside by the approximation of the pouches and clefts forms the six *pharyngeal or branchial* arches which extend from the primitive pharyngeal roof down to and across the pharyngeal floor to meet their fellows of the opposite side.

The early pharynx thus consists of a series of ridged arches and alternating grooves enclosing the pharyngeal lumen rather like a corrugated tube

lying between the developing brain dorsally and the heart ventrally. Each pharyngeal arch consists of a *mesodermal* core covered by endoderm on its internal surface and ectoderm on its external surface. As development proceeds each arch comes to contain the following elements:

1. An *artery* coming from the dorsal aorta and the aortic sac.
2. A *nerve* consisting of branches from sensory and motor ganglia such that each arch is supplied by a *specific* major nerve.
3. A *cartilage* bar.
4. A developing *muscle* mass.

The fate of the arch cartilages, the muscles which develop and the nerve of each arch are summarised in the following table (Table 14.1).

Development of the pharyngeal pouches

The four pharyngeal pouches lie between the pharyngeal arches and give rise to various organs and structures discussed below. That part of the fourth pouch which gives rise to the ultimobranchial body is sometimes described as a fifth pouch.

First pharyngeal pouch. The dorsal end of the first pharyngeal pouch deepens considerably forming the *tubotympanic recess*. A corresponding ingrowth of the first pharyngeal cleft results in the *endoderm* of the tubotympanic recess coming into contact with the *ectoderm* of the first pharyngeal cleft. The distal part of the tubotympanic recess widens, incorporates the ossicles which lie in the mesoderm above it, and eventually forms the middle ear cavity. The narrow proximal part forms the *pharyngotympanic tube*. The endodermal lining of the middle ear cavity together with the ectoderm of the pharyngeal cleft forms the *tympanic mem-*

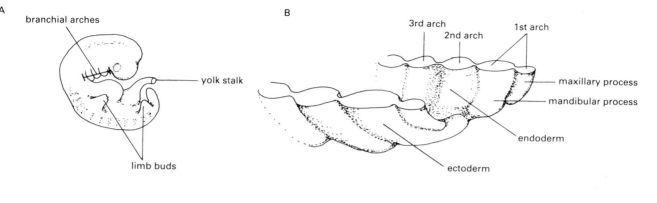

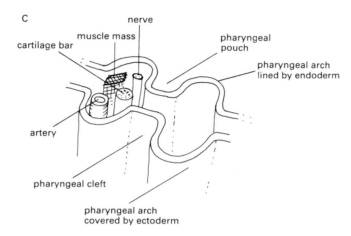

Fig. 14.1 Pharyngeal arches, clefts and pouches. A — Early embryo showing the pharyngeal (branchial) arches. B — Sectioned view along arches shown in A. The pharyngeal cavity is bounded on both sides by pharyngeal arches. C — Horizontal section through two adjacent arches to show a pharyngeal pouch, pharyngeal cleft and the contents of a pharyngeal arch.

Table 14.1 The fate of the arch cartilages and the muscles which develop from each pharyngeal arch

Arch	Cartilage	Fate of cartilage	Muscles	Nerve of arch
1	Meckel's	Malleus, incus, perichondrium persists as sphenomandibular ligament	Muscles of mastication, tensor tympani, tensor palati, mylohyoid, ant. belly of digastric	Trigeminal nerve (Vth cranial)
2	Reichert's	Stapes, styloid process, upper part of body of hyoid bone, perichondrium persists as stylohyoid ligament	Stapedius, stylohyoid, muscles of facial expression, post. belly of digastric	Facial nerve (VIIth cranial)
3		Lower part of hyoid bone	Stylopharyngeus	Glossopharyngeal nerve (IXth cranial)
4,6*		Cartilages fuse to form the thyroid, arytenoid, and cricoid cartilages of larynx	Cricothyroid, pharyngeal constrictors, intrinsic muscles of larynx	Vagus nerve — superior and recurrent laryngeal nerves (Xth cranial)

* the 5th arch is only transient in the human

brane and the first pharyngeal cleft forms the external auditory meatus.

Second pharyngeal pouch. The *palatine tonsil* develops from the lining of the second pouch. Endodermal cells of the pouch proliferate and form downgrowths into the underlying mesoderm. Lymphocytes accumulate around the endodermal downgrowths which eventually split to form crypts. The *supratonsillar cleft* in the fully formed tonsil is the persistent remnant of the second pouch.

The third and fourth pouches have a more complicated history and develop separate dorsal and ventral expansions.

Third pharyngeal pouch. The dorsal expansion of the third pouch forms the *inferior parathyroid gland*; its ventral expansion forms the epithelial component of the *thymus* gland. With development the thymus migrates caudally taking the inferior parathyroid gland with it. The bulk of the thymus fuses in the thorax with its counterpart from the opposite side, the tail eventually fragments and disappears. The inferior parathyroid gland comes to rest on the dorsal surface of the lower pole of the thyroid gland.

Fourth pharyngeal pouch. The dorsal expansion of the fourth pouch forms the *superior parathyroid gland*. The ventral expansion develops into the *ul-*

timobranchial body which fuses with the developing thyroid gland and forms the *parafollicular* ('C') cells of that gland.

Clinical considerations

1. Although the tail portion of the migrating thymus usually disappears, parts of it may persist as isolated areas of thymic tissue along its migratory track or can even be found imbedded within the thyroid gland.

2. The inferior parathyroid gland, although normally lying behind the thyroid gland near its lower pole, may be pulled into a lower position by the migrating thymus and be found within the thorax or, rarely, within the thymus itself.

DEVELOPMENT OF THE THYROID GLAND (Fig. 14.2)

The *thyroid* gland develops as a midline endodermal downgrowth in the pharyngeal floor between the first and second pharyngeal arches and comes into contact with the aortic sac. As this draws away from the pharynx the connection between the thyroid rudiment and the pharyngeal floor elongates forming the *thyroglossal duct*. The thyroid rudiment proliferates and forms two lobes united by an isthmus lying in front of the trachea. The bulk of the thyroglossal duct disappears, the site of its original attachment is marked by the *foramen caecum* on the tongue.

Clinical considerations

1. If some cells of the thyroglossal duct persist they may form *thyroglossal cysts*. These can be present, in the midline, at any point along the path of descent of the duct from the foramen caecum to the thyroid gland but about 50% lie in close relation to the hyoid bone. The cysts are soft and fluctuant and move upward on swallowing and on protrusion of the tongue.

2. Thyroglossal cysts are occasionally connected to the skin surface by midline *thyroglossal fistulae*. There may be discharge from such fistulae and they may become infected.

3. Aberrant masses of thyroid tissue, normally

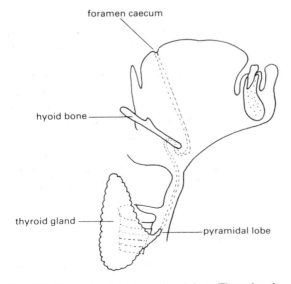

Fig. 14.2 The track of the thyroglossal duct. Thyroglossal duct cells may persist in the adult and give rise to cysts or aberrant masses of thyroid tissue.

quite functional, may be found at any point along the track of the thyroglossal duct but are most common in the posterior part of the tongue — the *lingual* thyroid. This may be large enough to obstruct the oropharynx.

4. The thyroid gland may descend beyond its normal position in the neck into the upper mediastinum forming a *retrosternal thyroid*.

5. An extra lobe of the thyroid — the *pyramidal lobe* — which develops from the lower part of the thyroglossal duct may be found projecting upwards from the isthmus.

6. A muscle, the *levator glandulae thyroideae*, is sometimes present passing from the hyoid to the thyroid isthmus. This marks the site of the lower part of the thyroglossal duct.

DEVELOPMENT OF THE TONGUE

The floor of the pharyngeal end of the foregut is formed by the ventral ends of the first, second and third pharyngeal arches which fuse in the midline.

The anterior part of the tongue develops from three thickenings of the ventral part of the first arch — the two *lateral lingual swellings* fusing with a median bud, the *tuberculum impar*. The posterior part of the tongue is formed by a median swelling of the third arch (forming part of the *hypobranchial eminence* or copula) growing forwards *over* the second arch to fuse with the three first arch processes which form the anterior portion of the tongue.

The line of fusion of the anterior and posterior parts of the tongue persists as the V-shaped *sulcus terminalis*. At its apex (which is directed posteriorly) the endoderm invades the underlying tissue to form the thyroglossal duct which proliferates downwards and, from its extremity, forms the thyroid gland. The site of the original downgrowth from which the thyroglossal duct developed remains on the tongue as the *foramen caecum*.

The sensory supply of the anterior part of the tongue is from the nerve of the first arch from which it derives — the mandibular branch of the trigeminal nerve. The sensory supply of the posterior part is from the nerve of the third arch — the glossopharyngeal nerve. Special sensory fibres of taste to the anterior part of the tongue are supplied by the facial nerve (chorda tympani branch) and to the posterior part of the tongue by the glossopharyngeal nerve.

The musculature of the tongue develops from myotomes which migrate from the occipital region and grow around the lateral pharyngeal wall to enter the developing tongue. The muscles arising from these myotomes are supplied by the hypoglossal nerve.

In the early stages of development the tongue is continuous with the rest of the tissues of the floor of the mouth. However, an ectodermal downgrowth gradually separates the tongue from the developing gingiva. This ectodermal downgrowth eventually disintegrates forming the linguogingival sulcus.

Clinical considerations

1. A congenitally short frenulum on the undersurface of the tongue may produce the condition known as 'tongue-tie'. This may interfere with normal suckling and, later, with speech but only rarely is surgical intervention necessary.

DEVELOPMENT OF THE SALIVARY GLANDS

The three main pairs of salivary glands all develop as outgrowths of stomatodeal ectoderm in the sixth and seventh weeks.

The *parotid* bud grows backwards from the inner aspect of the cheek toward the ear and later develops to form the acini and duct systems. As the gland develops, buccinator muscle surrounds the duct, which then comes to pierce it.

The *submandibular* bud develops on the floor of the mouth and grows backwards lateral to the tongue. The *sublingual* bud develops in a similar fashion at the side of the tongue.

Clinical considerations

1. A cystic swelling or *ranula*, due to obstruction of one or more of the sublingual ducts may be present at birth and interfere with normal suckling or become infected.

DEVELOPMENT OF THE RESPIRATORY TRACT

The respiratory tract appears as a midline *respiratory diverticulum* in the floor of the foregut caudal to the *epiglottic swelling* of the fourth arch. It deepens and is then separated from the foregut, except at the laryngeal entrance, by the growth of the *oesophagotracheal septum*. The laryngeal entrance or orifice is bounded anteriorly by the epiglottis and laterally by the arytenoid swellings. The laryngeal cartilages develop around this orifice.

The respiratory diverticulum continues to grow caudally forming the midline *trachea*. At its end two lateral outpocketings ramify to form the *lungs*. The foregut from which it has become separated forms the *oesophagus*.

Clinical considerations

1. Many abnormalities have been described in the respiratory tract ranging from complete *agenesis* of the lungs to ectopic lobes or abnormal divisions of the bronchial tree. Congenital *cysts* of the lung may be single or multiple, are usually symptomless, but may cause pressure on the rest of the lung or lobe, may rupture into the pleural cavity causing pneumothorax or become infected.

2. Oesophageal abnormalities also occur, the most common being *atresia* of the upper part of the oesophagus with the lower part being connected to the trachea by an *oesophagotracheal fistula*. Variations on this abnormality occur and prompt diagnosis is important since inhalation of fluids into the respiratory tree may occur.

DEVELOPMENT OF THE PHARYNGEAL CLEFTS

Of the pharyngeal clefts on the exterior surface of the developing embryo only the first is of developmental importance.

The dorsal end of the first cleft deepens and forms a blind sac which is directed inwardly toward the pharynx. With further development the ectodermal end of the sac comes in contact with the endodermal end of the corresponding first pharyngeal pouch which has grown outwards from the pharyngeal cavity. The exterior pouch forms the *external auditory meatus*. The ectodermal cells at the end of the cleft proliferate and form the *meatal plug*. This plug later disappears and the ectoderm at the end of the external auditory meatus participates in the formation of the eardrum.

On either side of the opening of the meatus small mesodermal proliferations, the *auricular hillocks*, appear and fuse to form the auricle of the ear.

Proliferation of the second arch mesoderm causes it to grow caudally and overlap the second, third and fourth clefts until it fuses with the *epipericardial ridge*. The buried clefts coalesce to form the *cervical sinus* which initially retains a connection with the exterior surface but eventually this is lost and the ectoderm forming the sinus walls disintegrates and the sinus disappears.

Clinical considerations (Fig. 14.3)

1. The cervical sinus, formed by the fusion of the buried second, third and fourth pharyngeal clefts, may persist forming a *branchial* or *lateral cervical cyst*, lined by squamous epithelium. These are often found just below the angle of the mandible

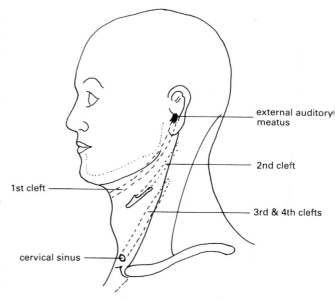

Fig. 14.3 The fate of the pharyngeal clefts. The 1st cleft persists as the external auditory meatus. Remnants of the other clefts may give rise to branchial cysts or fistula.

but may be present at any site along the anterior border of sternomastoid muscle. They are frequently filled with a pus-like fluid, rich in cholesterol.

2. The cervical sinus may remain in contact with the skin surface through a narrow *external branchial fistula* or, rarely, open into the pharynx in the tonsillar region (derived from the second pharyngeal pouch) through an *internal branchial fistula*. Internal and external branchial fistulae may coexist leading to a communication between the pharynx and the skin surface.

3. Fusion of the auricular hillocks is complex and many abnormalities of auricular development occur. One is the presence of *preauricular fistulae*

due to the persistence of a groove between hillocks.

4. The meatal plug of the first pharyngeal cleft may persist resulting in one form of congenital deafness.

DEVELOPMENT OF THE FACE (Fig. 14.4)

By the end of the fourth week of embryonic life the thin *bucco-pharyngeal membrane* which separates the stomatodeum from the early pharynx breaks down so that communication is established between the exterior and the pharyngeal end of the foregut.

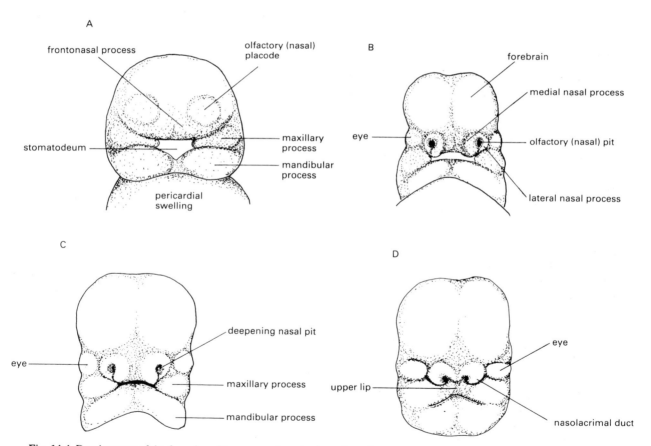

Fig. 14.4 Development of the face. A — The stomatodeum in the early embryo is bounded above by the frontonasal process, laterally by the maxillary processes and below by the mandibular processes. The buccopharyngeal membrane which separates the stomatodeum from the pharynx breaks down at an early stage. B — Development of the olfactory (nasal) pits. The developing eyes have moved forwards onto the face. C — The maxillary processes grow forwards on either side to fuse with the medial nasal and frontonasal processes and form the upper lip. The nasal pits continue to deepen. (See Fig. 14.5 for the fate of the nasal pits.) D — The upper lip has formed and the face has a human appearance. The cells forming the nasolacrimal furrow sink beneath the facial surface to form the nasolacrimal duct.

Mandibular processes derived from the ventral ends of the first branchial arches on each side grow around the embryo to meet and fuse in the midline immediately below the stomatodeal opening. Above the stomatodeal opening there is a mesodermal proliferation on the large bulge of the forebrain, forming a *frontonasal process*. On each side of this process the ectoderm thickens to form *olfactory placodes*. The medial and lateral edges of each placode become elevated forming *medial* and *lateral nasal processes*. The intervening tissue is now slightly depressed and is called the olfactory (nasal) pit.

Further proliferation from the cranial (upper) edge of the mandibular process on either side forms the *maxillary processes* which lie lateral to the stomatodeum. Each maxillary process grows around and above the stomatodeal opening and approaches the medial and lateral nasal processes, remaining separated from them, however, by well-defined grooves. Fusion occurs later. Formation of the upper lip in the region of the philtrum

is either derived from further medial growth of each maxillary process and fusion with its fellow of the opposite side and the medial nasal process above *or* by a downward growth of the medial nasal process to restrict the maxillary process contribution to the more lateral aspects of the lip. In either event, the *normal* formation of the upper lip requires the *co-ordinated* development and growth of three processes — the bilateral maxillary processes and the frontonasal process.

FORMATION OF THE NASAL CAVITY (Fig. 14.5)

As the developing head expands due to the rapid growth of the underlying brain the *nasal pits* elongate and become deep cavities. The entrance to each pit becomes clearly defined as the medial and lateral nasal processes increase in size forming a well-defined rim to the opening. Proliferation and

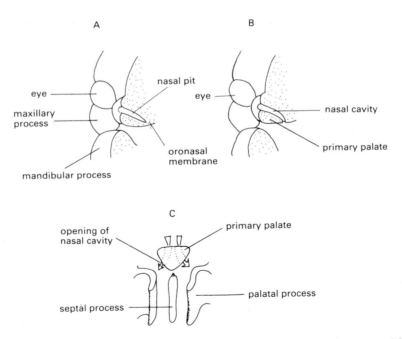

Fig. 14.5 Sagittal section through the nasal pit of one side. A — The nasal pit is deep but remains separated from the pharyngeal cavity by the oronasal membrane which is becoming progressively thinner. B — The oronasal membrane has broken down. The nasal pit now communicates with the pharynx (developing oral cavity) forming a nasal cavity. C — The roof of the developing oropharyngeal cavity. The formation of the early nasal cavities from the nasal pits gives rise to the primary palate. This will ultimately fuse with the palatal processes and the septal process to form the hard and soft palates. The nasal cavities will be therefore increased in size.

growth of the maxillary processes of either side toward the midline occurs and they fuse, first with the lateral nasal processes and then with the fronto-nasal processes. At this approximation of the *maxillary process* and the *lateral nasal process* the ectoderm thickens. This linear thickening runs from the medial aspect of the developing eye to the lateral side of the entrance to the nasal pit. The thickening gradually subsides below the surface as a solid cylinder of cells which eventually becomes canalised to form the *nasolacrimal duct* connecting the *lacrimal sac* to the nasal cavity. The paired entrances (nostrils) to the nasal cavities become separated from the stomatodeal opening by a clearly defined lip.

With further deepening of each nasal pit it becomes separated from the roof of the stomatodeum by a thin layer of tissue, the *oronasal membrane*. This disintegrates on either side so that each primitive nasal cavity now communicates directly with the stomatodeal cavity. The tissue lying between the nasal cavities and the anterior part of the stomatodeum in front of these openings is the *primary palate*. The tissue separating these early nasal cavities constitutes the *primary nasal septum*. The posterior ventral edge of the nasal septum grows backwards to await the elevation of the palatal processes to form the definitive palate.

Formation of the palate (Fig. 14.6)

The bulk of the early oral cavity (as defined above) is occupied by the *tongue* which has developed from the pharyngeal floor. As the anterior primary palate is being formed, inward and downwardly directed *palatal processes* develop from the inner aspect of each maxillary process. They are prevented from reaching the midline by the great mass of the tongue but with further growth of the embryo the tongue descends and physicochemical changes in the palatal processes cause them to elevate and extend rapidly to meet in the midline forming the *secondary palate*. Anteriorly the palatal processes are opposed to the back of the primary palate. The *incisive foramen* marks the midline between the primary and secondary palates. In the midline the palatal processes meet each other and the lower edge of the nasal septum which projects down from the roof of the cavity. These processes

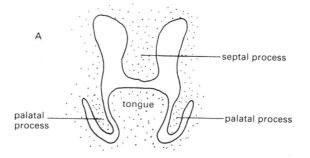

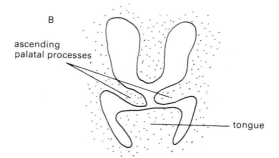

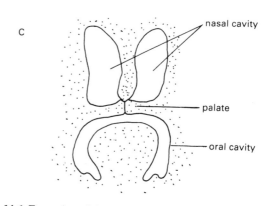

Fig. 14.6 Formation of the palate. Coronal section through the developing nasal and oral cavities. A — The palatal processes lie on either side of the tongue. B — Elevation of the palatal processes to meet the septal process. C — Fusion of the palatal and septal processes. The endodermal covering of the processes breaks down and fusion of the mesoderm takes place. Epithelial remnants persist and can give rise to epithelial cysts.

now fuse from before backwards by disintegration of the intervening epithelium.

The hard and soft palates therefore require the co-ordinated fusion of the maxillary and fronto-nasal processes (upper lip and primary palate), the nasal septum and palatal processes.

Position of the eye

The eyes develop initially on the sides of the head and gradually move from this lateral position onto the front of the face. By the eight week of embryonic life the face, oral and nasal cavities are formed and the embryo has assumed a more human appearance.

Clinical considerations (Fig. 14.7)

The development of the face and palate by growth and eventual fusion of the processes is complex and developmental defects, mainly cleft deformities, are common. These are frequently associated with other congenital conditions and it is good practice to make a search for these also.

Cleft deformities of the face and palate can be divided into two categories, the *anterior* and *posterior* cleft deformities, with the *incisive foramen* as the dividing landmark. Anterior cleft deformities are caused by a failure in fusion of the *medial nasal* and *maxillary* processes. Posterior cleft deformities

are caused by a failure in fusion of the *palatal* processes.

Incidence and causation

The incidence of these deformities varies with their site, for instance, clefts of the lip (a type of anterior cleft), with or without a concomitant cleft palate, occur in about 1 in 1000 births. They are more common in the male and in certain races. Clefts of the palate *only* occur more rarely (about 1 in 2500 births) and are more common in girls. It has been shown that fusion of the palatal shelves in the female occurs later than in the male and this may explain the greater frequency with which this defect occurs in the female. The incidence of cleft lip increases with increasing maternal age, the incidence of cleft palate does not.

In both defects, in families in which a parent, a relative or a previous sibling has a cleft, the likelihood of another child having a similar defect is increased, although inheritance in a dominant, recessive or simple Mendelian form is unlikely. Experimentally, a variety of agents can produce cleft palate in animals but no single factor has been implicated in man. Although it is not yet clear, the causation of facial cleft deformities is probably multifactorial and influenced by many genetic and environmental factors.

Mechanisms

Possible mechanisms of cleft formation may be:
1. Persistence of the epithelium on the opposing surfaces of the processes which prevents union of their mesoderm.
2. Failure of sufficient penetration of mesoderm into the area of fusion resulting in the breakdown of the unsupported area and the formation of a cleft.
3. Malalignment of the processes.
4. Disruption of the area by traction forces — this may account for the bands of connective tissue which are occasionally found traversing a cleft lip.

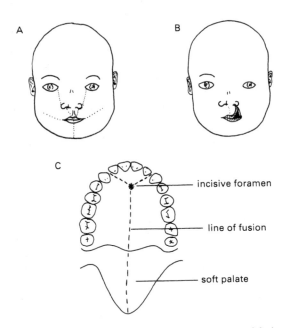

Fig. 14.7 Development of the face. A — The lines of fusion of the processes which make up the face. Facial clefts can occur along one or more of these lines. B — Hare-lip results due to the failure of fusion of the maxillary and frontonasal processes. It may be restricted to the lip but may be complicated by cleft of the palate. C — The lines of fusion of the processes making up the hard and soft palates.

Types of cleft

A. Anterior clefts. 1. *Median cleft lip* is a rare anomaly due to failure of development of the philtrum by fusion in the midline. It may occur in conjunction with a midline cleft of the nose.

2. *Cleft lip.* Clefts of the lip usually lie to the side of the philtrum and may vary in severity. The defect may be confined to a slight notching of the red margin of the lip but may be more severe with the cleft extending into the nostril on the affected side. This leads to widening of this nostril with flattening of the ala. In 15% of cases the clefts are bilateral.

3. *Cleft lip and primary palate.* In more severe cases the cleft lip is associated with a cleft in the alveolar process of the maxilla between the lateral incisor and the canine teeth, and this may extend backwards to the incisive foramen. A defect of this nature may occur bilaterally with complete separation between the primary and secondary palates and in such cases the primary palate (premaxilla) may be displaced anteriorly.

4. A *facial cleft* is a rare anomaly in which the anterior cleft extends upwards beside the nose to the medial corner of the eye, usually exposing the nasolacrimal duct to the surface. The defect is caused by a failure of fusion between the *lateral nasal* and the *maxillary* processes of the affected side.

5. *Cleft lower lip* occurs rarely and may be associated with a cleft mandible and tongue. It is caused by failure of fusion of the mandibular processes in the midline.

B. *Posterior clefts.* 1. The least severe deformity of this type is the *cleft uvula* which is of minimal clinical significance.

2. *Cleft palate.* More severely, the cleft may involve a failure of fusion of the whole of the secondary palate behind the incisive foramen. Clinically this is termed a *partial* cleft of the palate.

3. Anterior and posterior clefts may coexist to form the clinically-termed *complete* cleft of the palate in which both the secondary and the primary palates are involved. This may occur bilaterally with separation of the primary palate from the secondary palate *and* the secondary palatal shelves from each other.

Management of clefts

Clefts of the lip and palate may present problems in feeding of the infant, depending on their se-

verity, and uncorrected defects can lead to severe speech disorders as well as being cosmetically unsatisfactory. Isolated clefts of the lip usually present no great difficulties in feeding and are surgically corrected, if possible, in the early months of life.

Clefts of the palate, however, can present feeding problems with inability to suckle and regurgitation of feed into the nasal cavity. Infections of the nasopharynx and the middle ear may then occur. Such infants may have to be fed by spoon or gastric tube. Surgical repair is usually carried out at about one year of age so that normal speech can develop. Delay may lead to speech defects which require intensive therapy. Surgical repair usually produces excellent results and coordination between surgeon, orthodontist and speech therapist is important in achieving normal or near-normal function.

Other conditions

1. *Development cysts.* The epithelium on the surfaces of the facial swellings disintegrates and disappears prior to their fusion. Incomplete disappearance may lead to the development of epithelial-lined cysts termed *inclusion dermoids* along the lines of fusion of the processes. They may be situated in various sites, for example:

a. *External angular dermoid*: found in the lateral part of the eyebrow.

b. *Midline dermoid*: situated in the floor of the mouth between the mandibular processes.

c. *Epithelial pearls*: found along the lines of fusion of the palate.

d. *Developmental cysts of jaw*: arise along the lines of fusion of the developing maxilla and mandible. The commonest is the *globulomaxillary* cyst between the premaxilla and the maxilla and lying between the upper lateral incisor and canine teeth.

2. *Macro- and microstomia.* Macrostomia is an unusually large opening of the mouth which results from failure of the mandibular and maxillary processes to fuse properly at the corners of the mouth. Microstomia, as its name implies, results from excessive fusion of the selfsame processes producing an unusually small opening of the mouth.

Radiology

X-rays and visible light are both part of the electromagnetic spectrum and have similar properties. Both can produce an image when a photographic emulsion is exposed to them, but X-rays, having a shorter wavelength, have the ability to penetrate solid objects, such as the human body, and can therefore give rise to an image of its underlying structure.

The degree of penetration of X-rays depends on their absorption by the body tissues. Structures which are less dense, e.g. air, air-containing structures such as the lungs and paranasal sinuses, fat and the soft tissues, allow a greater penetration of X-rays and are relatively *radiolucent*. Denser structures, such as bone and teeth, allow less penetration; and metallic objects, such as dental fillings, surgical implants and foreign bodies may block X-rays totally. Such structures are relatively, or totally, *radio-opaque*.

The relative radiolucency or radio-opacity of the tissues produces different images on the developed radiographic film. Radio-opaque structures, with little X-ray penetration, appear as white areas; radiolucent structures, with a greater X-ray penetration, appear as black areas on the developed film.

TYPES OF X-RAY PHOTOGRAPH

X-rays may be used in a variety of ways to produce different types of image of the body tissues.

Commonest is the *radiograph*, in which X-rays are directed through the stationary subject onto a stationary film. The image produced is, of course, a two-dimensional representation of a three-dimensional object and the fact that superimposition of the images of structures therefore occurs must always be borne in mind when such films are interpreted.

Obviously, a large variety of images can be produced, depending on the angle at which the subject is positioned relative to the X-ray beam and to the photographic plate. The common standard views of the skull and facial bones will be discussed later.

The denser, or more radio-opaque, structures show up well in standard radiographs but most soft tissue structures are not well illustrated and a variety of procedures are available to make their radiographic visualisation easier.

Certain soft tissue structures can be highlighted by the use of radio-opaque *contrast media*. Such media may be injected into the arterial system of an area to produce *arteriograms*, into the venous system to produce *venograms* and into the lymphatic vessels to produce *lymphangiograms*. Cranial arteriography may help in the visualisation of arterial disease, e.g. arteriosclerosis, aneurysm, arteriovenous malformation; in congenital malformation, e.g. absent or aberrant vessels, stenosis, 'berry' aneurysm; in neoplasia by illustrating new vessel formation; and in neoplastic or other intracranial space-occupying lesions by illustrating the displacement of vessels from their normal sites.

The ducts of glands or organs may be cannulated and outlined by the injection of a radio-opaque medium, as in *sialography* of the major salivary glands, cholecystography of the biliary tree and retrograde pyelography of the genitourinary tract.

A hollow viscus may be outlined by the insertion

or ingestion of medium, e.g. barium swallow, meal and enema outlining the gastrointestinal tract or a bronchogram outlining the bronchial tree.

There are numerous other uses of contrast media in the visualisation of otherwise poorly seen structures.

The superimposition of images, especially on radiographs of the skull with its complex bony arrangement, may mask an area of interest. However, in *tomography*, X-rays can be 'focussed' on a slice through the subject at a specific depth, by moving the film and the X-ray source in opposite directions during the exposure. The resulting film shows focused images at the desired depth and blurred images of structures lying superficial or deep to this plane.

Another means of producing a focused image in a desired plane is by *computerised axial tomography* or *CT scanning*. In this technique, a narrow-beam X-ray source traverses the area to be scanned in the desired plane, rotating through 1° after each traverse until it has completed a semicircle. Density detectors mounted opposite the source measure the density during each traverse and the computer mathematically reconstructs the density measurements to give a representation of density for each point within that plane. The final image is produced on a cathode ray tube and can be recorded as a Polaroid photograph. A series of cuts is usually made through successive planes of the area.

The movements which occur within joints or the passage of contrast medium through a soft-tissue structure may be illustrated by using a fluorescent screen rather than a radiographic film. Radiographs may be taken at desired intervals to provide a record. Fluoroscopy is of great value in the introduction and positioning of cardiac catheters and external pacemakers into the appropriate chambers of the heart.

RADIOGRAPHS OF THE SKULL AND FACIAL BONES

General considerations

The X-ray beam emanates from a 'point' source and the beam is therefore divergent. Structures which lie close to the film will show the least mag-

nification, those furthest from the film will be correspondingly larger.

Terms

Posteroanterior (PA) radiographs are produced by positioning the X-ray source posteriorly and the radiographic film anteriorly and directing the X-ray beam from the posterior to the anterior aspect of the subject. Anteriorly-placed structures show least magnification and their image is clearer.

Anteroposterior (AP) radiographs are produced by directing the X-ray beam in the opposite direction to PA radiographs, from anterior to posterior. Posteriorly-placed structures are least magnified and clearer.

Lateral radiographs are of two types. In a *right lateral* radiograph the right side of the subject is placed nearest the film. The image of left-sided

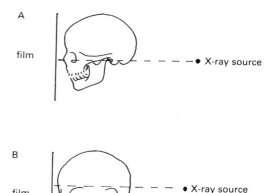

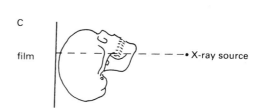

Fig. 15.1 Positioning of head relative to X-ray source. A — Posteroanterior projection (PA). B — Left lateral projection. C — Submentovertex projection.

structures is enlarged and superimposed upon the smaller, clearer image of right-sided structures. *Left lateral* radiographs are produced in a similar fashion, with the opposite result.

Many other radiographic positions are, of course, in common use. Most are *oblique* projections of one form or another in which the subject is positioned relative to the X-ray source and the radiographic film in such a way as to highlight a particular area or structure by avoiding the superimposition of other structures as much as possible.

Radiographs of the skull (Fig. 15.1)

The four standard radiographic views of the skull are:

1. A posteroanterior (PA) projection.
2. A right and left lateral projection.
3. An anteroposterior (AP or Towne's) projection.
4. A basal projection.

1. In a PA radiograph of the skull the subject is positioned so that the *midsagittal* line and the *canthomeatal* line (from the outer canthus of the eye to the external auditory meatus) both lie perpendicular to the radiographic film. The X-ray beam is directed so that its centre passes through the midline of the head in the canthomeatal plane, centred on the nasion, and strikes the film perpendicularly.

In a radiograph of this type the anterior wall of the skull vault, the frontal and ethmoidal sinuses, the crista galli and nasal septum and the upper parts of the orbital margins are well visualised. The lower parts of the orbital margins are obscured by the shadow of the petrous parts of the temporal bones. This can be avoided and the whole orbital margin outlined clearly by a modified view in which the subject is positioned as before, the X-ray beam remains centred on the nasion but its angle is now directed caudally by 20°. This projects the shadows of the petrous bones clear of the orbits.

2. In right and left lateral radiographs the subject is positioned so that the midsagittal line is parallel to the radiographic film and the beam is directed through the centre of the temporal area on a line through the forehead 1 cm or so above the eyebrows.

The pituitary fossa, anterior and posterior clinoid processes, the floor of the anterior cranial fossa, the meningeal markings, the coronal and lambdoid sutures and the parietal and squamous temporal bones are well visualised in these radiographs. Much of the middle cranial fossa is obscured by the shadow of the bulk of the petrous bones. Occasionally, this radio-opaque block is pierced by a circular lucency, marking the site of the external auditory meatus.

Parts of the sphenoid and maxillary sinuses and the posterior cranial fossa can be seen, as well as the ramus and body of each side of the mandible superimposed upon one another.

3. The AP radiograph is produced by positioning the subject so that the midsagittal and canthomeatal lines lie perpendicular to the film. The X-ray beam is then directed anteroposteriorly on a line through the external auditory meatus, tilted 30° or so caudally.

The foramen magnum, occipital area and lambdoid suture are well visualised on this view.

4. In the basal (basilar, submentovertical) view the subject is positioned so that the midsagittal line is perpendicular to the film. The X-ray beam is directed from below the chin, between the angles of the mandible, to the vertex of the skull perpendicular to the canthomeatal line.

The foramen magnum and certain other basal foramina and the sphenoid sinuses are well visualised. The mandible, maxillary sinuses and zygomatic arches can also be seen on this view.

Radiographs of the facial bones

Although the midfacial bones can be evaluated to some degree in the standard skull views certain specialised projections give better views of this area, namely:

1. The *Water's erect* view, in which the subject is positioned with the midsagittal line perpendicular to the film and the canthomeatal line tilted upwards at 45° to bring the chin and the nose into contact with the film. In this manner the orbital floor lies perpendicular to the film and in the radiograph its shadow is visible below the shadow of the inferior orbital margin.

Isolated fractures of the orbital floor ('blow-out' fractures) can be identified more clearly in this view than in the standard P.A. skull radiograph. Also seen clearly in this view is the maxillary sinus with its roof, medial and lateral walls. The sinus may be opaque or show a fluid-level due to the presence of pus or mucus in infections or allergic conditions or blood following trauma. The orbital margin, frontal sinus, nasal septum, zygomaticofrontal suture and part of the zygomatic arch are also clearly seen.

Fractures of the zygomatic complex can be recognised on the Water's view. This so-called 'quadripod' fracture consists of the following findings: a fracture of the inferior orbital margin and orbital floor, fracture of the lateral wall of the maxillary sinus, opening of the zygomaticofrontal suture and fracture of the zygomatic arch. The maxillary antrum may be opaque due to a haematoma into it following trauma.

2. *Occipitomental (10° and 30°)* views are taken with the subject positioned as for the erect Water's view but with the X-ray beam tilted at 10° and 30° caudally and centred on the occipital bone 3 cm above the external occipital protuberance.

These views show the maxillary sinuses clearly by removing the superimposition of the petrous bone shadows.

Lateral views, with the X-ray beam centred through the maxillary sinus, are useful in conjunction with the facial views described above but are of less value since the sinuses are superimposed upon one another. The nasal bones are seen clearly in appropriate lateral radiographs.

Other views are also available which can demonstrate certain aspects of the midfacial bones, including occlusal views of the maxilla and intraoral views of desired areas. Such radiographs are of great value in the diagnosis of dental disease such as caries and root abscess and conditions such as tooth impaction. Tangential views of the zygomatic arch may demonstrate depressed fractures of this structure, although uncommon in isolation.

Other facial radiographs include radiographs to demonstrate particular paranasal sinuses, the petrous temporal bone, mastoid air cells and the optic foramen. Tomography is occasionally of great value in demonstrating lesions of the maxillary sinus walls, and the advent of CT scanning is proving of great use in the radiographic investigation of the orbit and paranasal sinuses.

Radiographs of the mandible and TM joints

Routinely, three radiographs are necessary for an evaluation of the mandible. More specialised views may be requested subsequently for a more accurate or clearer representation of specific lesions or areas of interest.

1. A *posteroanterior* (PA or 'horseshoe') view demonstrates the body, the angles and part of the rami of the mandible. The condylar head is not visualised due to the superimposition of the mastoid processes. The subject is positioned with the midsagittal and canthomeatal lines perpendicular to the film. The X-ray beam passes posteroanteriorly through the subject perpendicular to the film and centred on the lips.

2. Right and left *oblique lateral* views are taken with the subject positioned so that the midsagittal line is parallel to the film. The X-ray beam is tilted cranially by 45° and directed from a point midway between the angle of one side and the symphysis to the angle of the opposite side. This eliminates the superimposition of the mandibular bodies, angles and rami and gives a clear view of the body, angle, ramus and condylar neck of the mandible on the side nearest the film.

3. The *reverse (PA) Towne's* projection (see Radiographs of the skull) is used to demonstrate the condylar necks of the mandible, not clearly visualised in the standard P.A. mandibular view.

Intraoral and occlusal views can also be performed on desired areas of the mandible and the TM joints may be visualised using *lateral TM joint* (Schuller) views in which the subject is positioned with the midsagittal line parallel to the film and the X-ray beam tilted 30° caudally and centred on the external auditory meatus of the side nearest the radiographic plate. Views can be taken with the mouth open and closed to demonstrate joint function and range of movement or dislocation of the joint. Tomography of the TM joint may also be useful in demonstrating intracapsular lesions.

Orthopantomography, in which a panorama of the maxilla and mandible and their teeth is produced by rotating an X-ray source around the subject, may occasionally be of value in locating abnormalities. The radiograph produced by this technique is usually not as informative as those produced by the standard techniques discussed above, but it is of value for its speed and for general recording purposes.

VIEWING THE RADIOGRAPH

Radiographs should be viewed against an appropriate coldlight illuminator. A more powerful light source may be needed to visualise fine detail in some areas. The habit of viewing radiographs by natural light from a window or by the light from any other than the recommended sources is strongly discouraged.

The radiograph should be viewed in its correct position, as if one was looking at a patient.

Each radiograph should be interpreted in a systematic fashion and, in structures which are present bilaterally, sides should be compared.

As an example, in the PA skull radiograph, note:

1. If the positioning is correct by the presence or absence of rotation and deviation of the midline:

2. The shape, size and symmetry of the skull vault and the thickness of its bones:

3. The position, presence or absence of the visible sutures, the sagittal, lambdoid and parts of the coronal sutures:

4. Trace the orbital margins, noting the presence of any discontinuity or 'step':

5. Examine the frontal and ethmoidal sinuses and the visible parts of the maxillary sinuses, noting any opacity within them, the presence of any fluid-level or disruption to their walls:

6. The extent of the nasal cavities and any septal deviation.

7. Trace the mandibular rami and lower borders:

8. Check the number, position and occlusion of the teeth:

9. Examine the bones of the vault for markings of meningeal vessels and diploic veins, fractures or areas of cortical discontinuity, areas of radiolucency or density and, if the pineal gland is calcified, whether it is deviated from the midline.

A systematic observation should be made of all radiographs.

Having a dried anatomical skull to hand is of great help in the understanding of radiographs of the skull and facial bones (Figs 15.2, 15.3, 15.4).

In the investigation of head injuries, particularly those caused by road traffic accidents, radiographs of the cervical spine should be requested routinely since injuries, e.g. 'whiplash' injuries, may have been inflicted to this area as well as to the skull vault and facial bones.

Figs 15.2, 15.3, 15.4
Radiographs of a disarticulated anatomical skull. Examination of radiographs and their associated skull is extremely helpful in understanding and interpreting radiographs.

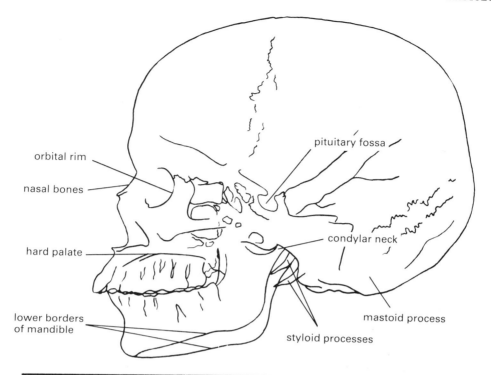

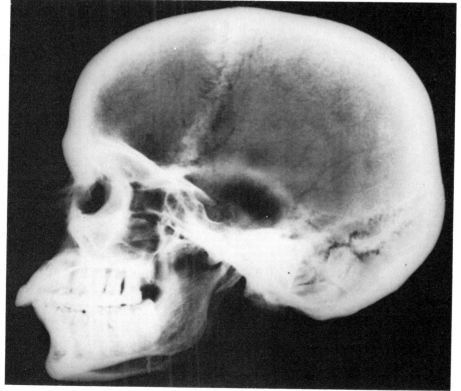

Fig. 15.2 Lateral view of skull. The styloid processes in this skull are extremely long.

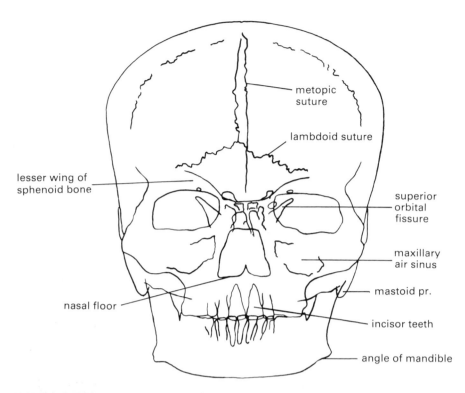

- metopic suture
- lambdoid suture
- lesser wing of sphenoid bone
- superior orbital fissure
- maxillary air sinus
- nasal floor
- mastoid pr.
- incisor teeth
- angle of mandible

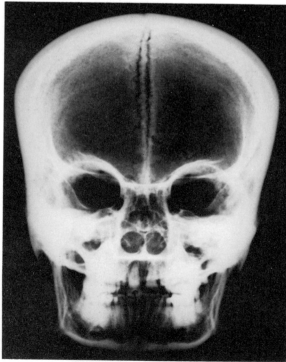

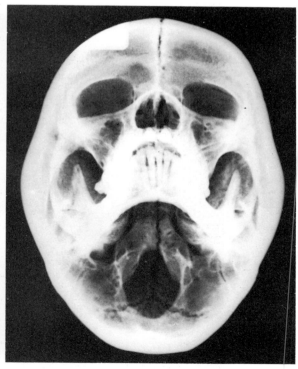

Fig. 15.3 PA view of skull. The metopic suture has not fused in this skull.

Fig. 15.4 Occipitomental view of skull. This view is particularly valuable for the facial bones.

Index